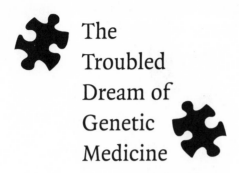

The
Troubled
Dream of
Genetic
Medicine

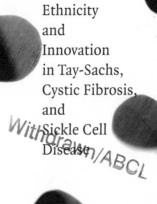

Ethnicity
and
Innovation
in Tay-Sachs,
Cystic Fibrosis,
and
Sickle Cell
Disease

The
Troubled
Dream of
Genetic
Medicine

KEITH
WAILOO
AND
STEPHEN
PEMBERTON

THE JOHNS HOPKINS UNIVERSITY PRESS Baltimore

© 2006 The Johns Hopkins University Press
All rights reserved. Published 2006
Printed in the United States of America on acid-free paper
9 8 7 6 5 4 3 2 1

The Johns Hopkins University Press
2715 North Charles Street
Baltimore, Maryland 21218-4363
www.press.jhu.edu

Library of Congress Cataloging-in-Publication Data
Wailoo, Keith.
The troubled dream of genetic medicine : ethnicity and
innovation in Tay-Sachs, cystic fibrosis, and sickle cell
disease / Keith Wailoo and Stephen Pemberton.
     p. ; cm.
Includes bibliographical references and index.
ISBN 0-8018-8325-3 (hard cover : alk. paper) —
ISBN 0-8018-8326-1 (pbk. : alk. paper)
1. Genetic disorders—Research—Moral and ethical
aspects. 2. Ethnic groups—Diseases. 3. Tay-Sachs
disease—Genetic aspects. 4. Cystic fibrosis—Genetic
aspects. 5. Sickle cell anemia—Genetic aspects.
I. Pemberton, Stephen Gregory. II. Title.
[DNLM: 1. Genetic Diseases, Inborn—ethnology.
2. Genetic Diseases, Inborn—prevention & control.
3. Anemia, Sickle Cell. 4. Cystic Fibrosis. 5. Health
Services Accessibility. 6. Tay-Sachs Disease.
QZ 50 W139t 2006]
RB155.5.W35 2006
616'.042—dc22   2005021184

A catalog record for this book is available from the British
Library.

CONTENTS

ACKNOWLEDGMENTS

This book is the product of an extended collaboration between the authors. It grew out of a study of the complex issues raised by gene therapy—a project funded by the Ethical, Legal, and Social Issues (ELSI) Research Program of the National Human Genome Research Institute. Many people share credit for helping this investigation evolve into its current form. In the initial stages, our ELSI co-investigators at the University of North Carolina Chapel Hill provided crucial insight. We are especially indebted to Larry Churchill and Nancy King in the Department of Social Medicine and Myra Collins in the Department of Pathology.

Since those beginnings, the book has evolved thanks to the support of two extraordinary organizations. The James S. McDonnell Foundation Centennial Fellowship in the History of Science awarded to Keith Wailoo in 1999 helped expand the scope of the work by fitting the stories of cystic fibrosis, Tay-Sachs, and sickle cell disease into the broader context of racial politics, pain, and the politics of biomedicine in twentieth-century America. The McDonnell Fellowship underwrote a series of cross-disciplinary workshops on these topics and allowed the authors to continue their collaboration in their moves from the University of North Carolina to new positions at Rutgers, the State University of New Jersey. A Robert Wood Johnson Investigator Award in Health Policy for Keith Wailoo furthered those dimensions of this research dealing with problems of ethnicity, race, and pain.

Together, the McDonnell Foundation and the Robert Wood Johnson Foundation helped create a rich research environment in which the energies and insights of many colleagues and research assistants were brought to the cultural study of disease and the biomedical sciences. Sincere thanks to the following research assistants: Ann Kakaliourous, Reggie Pearson, Moshe Usadi, and

Rachel Watkins at UNC; and Curt Cardwell, Joseph Gabriel, Carolina Giraldo, William Gordon, Justin Lorts, Rachel McLaughlin, Richard Mizelle, Khalil Muhammad, Dominique Padurano, Jane Park, Stefani Pfeiffer, Michele Rotunda, Lauren Waxman, and Christine Zemla at Rutgers.

Many others provided valuable commentary on individual chapters or crucial suggestions regarding the book as a whole. At an early stage, Allan Brandt and Michael Knowles offered key insights, and Charles Rosenberg and Julie Livingston were astute readers as the book evolved. When the project neared completion, we benefited from the valuable critique and suggestions of Gerald Grob, Alison Isenberg, Jay Kaufman, Samantha Kelly, David Mechanic, Sandy Sufian, and Moshe Usadi. Editorial guidance from Jacqueline Wehmueller at the Johns Hopkins University Press, as well as the expert advice of copy editor Mary Yates and two outside readers, extended the range and clarity of the book.

Finally, hearty thanks to Keith Wailoo's colleagues in the Institute for Health, Health Care Policy, and Aging Research and in the Department of History at Rutgers, New Brunswick, and to Stephen Pemberton's colleagues in the Federated Department of History at the New Jersey Institute of Technology and Rutgers, Newark, for creating the intellectually vibrant communities in which this project flourished.

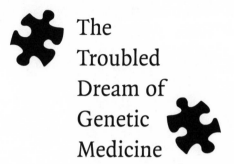

The
Troubled
Dream of
Genetic
Medicine

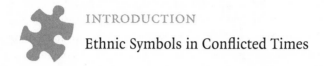

Ethnic Symbols in Conflicted Times

Why do controversies over race become attached, as they often do, to discussions of modern genetics? How do innovations in genetics and medicine become entangled with problems of ethnicity and disease disparities across groups? This book offers answers and historical perspective on the frequent collision between medical innovation and problems of race and ethnicity in America.

For better or worse, tensions between innovation and ethnicity have been with us for decades, and they have been a particularly potent force in the histories of three diseases and the people most often afflicted by them: Tay-Sachs disease (TSD) and Jewish Americans, cystic fibrosis (CF) and Caucasians, and sickle cell disease (SCD) and African Americans.[1] These three diseases are much more than personal crises; they are topics of biological fascination and crucibles of social debate. And for American society at large their stories frame broad questions about the meaning of race and ethnicity, about the promise of innovation, about the ability of diverse groups to shape healthy futures for themselves, and about who among us believes in the promise of the coming genetics revolution, who demurs, and who is best positioned to benefit from it. At one time or another each malady has stood out as an exemplary racial or ethnic concern while also representing the promise of genetic medicine. At frequent intervals over the years, technical discussions about these diseases—about their prevention, detection, and treatment—have spiraled into broader social controversies. And so, in the stories of these diseases we can see the fault lines and divisions in American society itself.

As we enter the age of genetic medicine, increasing knowledge of the human genome and genetic diseases thrusts new dilemmas of technology, ethics, and social justice into the public spotlight with increasing urgency.[2] At every turn, new therapies and diagnostic advances emerge and the possibility of conquering disease comes into view. Media reports and professional studies recite the promise in a steady drumbeat. Genetics in our time will have powerful implications for all humanity. Already, certain tests (such as tests for the breast cancer genes BRCA1 and BRCA2) hold out the possibility of identifying high-risk genes carried in people's bodies, genes that decades later may produce cancer. Such tests promise all Americans that early action may prevent the disease, but they also raise unsettling ethical and social dilemmas across a diverse nation.

Different people—women, men, physicians, entrepreneurs, and members of diverse ethnic groups—take the promise of genetic medicine to mean different things. For women who test positive for BRCA1 and BRCA2, for example, preventive mastectomy has become one of the most controversial options. Not surprisingly, physicians and ethicists are troubled by such choices, perplexed by the idea of removing healthy breasts because of a gene associated with a "risk" of future disease. At the same time, entrepreneurs have generated a great deal of hype about the gene therapy enterprise, which was once described as "bottling the stuff of dreams." As early as 1985, headlines in *Business Week* were suggesting that "gene doctors [were] on the verge of curing life's cruelest diseases."[3] But here too the results have been mixed, and the implications have been varied. Different groups have responded to the hype differently—some regarding the entrepreneurs, the venture capitalists, and the high expectations with suspicion, others wholeheartedly embracing the promise of breakthrough medicine. These differences are rooted in profoundly divergent cultural perspectives about technology, business, and the promise of innovation—perspectives that overlap in compelling ways with ideologies of race and ethnicity. What accounts for the different kinds of promises made by boosters of genetic medicine to African Americans, Jewish Americans, and Anglo-Americans? What accounts for the different ways in which diverse groups have perceived the hype, interpreted the message, and experienced the effects of the genetics revolution? As genetic medicine continually pushes into new terrain, there is a pressing need to study the moment and chart a course that recognizes the risks and rewards of these innovations for Americans across a wide social spectrum.[4]

Such questions, considered historically, take us to the heart of vexing controversies in race and ethnicity. How could Linus Pauling, one of the pioneers of the genetics revolution, suggest in the late 1960s that "there should be tattooed on the forehead of every young person a symbol showing possession of the sickle-cell gene or whatever similar gene"? How could Francis Collins, the director of the National Human Genome Project, in the early 1990s characterize an Ultra-Orthodox Jewish plan to prevent births of babies with Tay-Sachs disease, cystic fibrosis, and other genetic diseases as a "moderate nightmare" when only a few years earlier many experts had hailed similar programs as successful models?[5] And what did it mean for the genetics revolution that each of these diseases had a racial cast and that cystic fibrosis was widely discussed as a "Caucasian disease" at the same time that gene therapy was emerging as a powerful dream?[6] Such questions lie at the heart of this book. The answers shed light on the role of race in modern genetics and the sweeping cultural meanings attached to genetic medicine in our time.

Why place these three diseases at the center of the story of modern genetic medicine? In the mind-set of modern genetic medicine, Tay-Sachs disease, cystic fibrosis, and sickle cell disease are related to each other in one way: they are all hereditary diseases, passed from parents to offspring by a similar process of transmission.[7] This similarity has allowed many people to regard them as parallel maladies, leading even scientists to think that efforts to treat them should have a common focus: a gene-based strategy of cure. But the similarity ends there, because these maladies also have strikingly different biological, social, and cultural profiles. The first disorder, TSD, is a rapidly degenerative, invariably fatal childhood disorder that has come to be associated with Jews of Ashkenazic descent. CF is a malady with higher life expectancy, but it is still often deadly and has come to be associated with Caucasian people of European descent. Finally, SCD is a disease associated with recurrent pain and high childhood mortality in people of African descent. Efforts to manage these diseases have resulted in diverse social controversies, each reflecting much about the group involved and about specific aspects of illness as experienced by patients, their families, and their communities. In the case of TSD, the suffering of children and parents has often been understood against a broader backdrop of Ashkenazic Jewish history and of Jewish suffering and survival: in the early 1980s, for example, one brochure warning Jewish parents about TSD was "printed in blue and white, the colors of the Jewish prayer shawl and of the flag of Israel." [8] Against such a powerful cultural backdrop, it becomes easy to grasp how genetic information can become entangled with the survival of communities. The histories of CF and white people and of SCD as an important African-American concern follow quite different trajectories, and yet they too suggest the potent links between disease, genetic knowledge, and group identity. [9]

As these case histories make clear, genetic medicine is neither monolithic nor uniform. It emerges in diverse arenas, carried out by a wide array of specialists: neurologists in TSD, pulmonologists in CF, and hematologists in SCD, as well as oncologists, surgeons, and many others. Each specialty group, as we shall see, has its own agendas for putting genetics to use. Each has pursued the business opportunities of genetic medicine in different ways, and each has developed its own sensibilities about the cultural issues surrounding these diseases and the groups affected by them. One hematologist in 2003 could portray the hype surrounding imminent cures as a disservice to sickle cell patients, while a pediatric pulmonary disease specialist working with cystic fibrosis patients could promise in 1992 that "in the next decade, we are going to see a revolution in the treatment for this disease."[10] Such professional diversity has shaped not only the histories of these diseases but also cultural ideas about the promise of genetics. To understand these diverse investments, one must look closely at the practitioners who rally around these diseases, at their interests and professional debates, at their therapeutic conundrums, and at the social, ethical, and economic issues that have confronted them as well as patients and families.

The hype surrounding innovations like gene therapy is fueled by a powerful notion that has defined American medicine for much of the past century: the notion that we are always on the verge of a major breakthrough in the treatment of deadly disease. The cases examined here are replete with variations on this recurring theme, gene therapy being only the most recent chapter of the familiar drama. We evaluate the promise of "breakthrough" medicines, and a wide range of other sensibilities about the genetics revolution, by looking closely at how innovations have performed in past struggles against disease. How is it that antibiotics could one day be at the forefront of the battle against cystic fibrosis yet only a few years later be perceived as a profound problem for CF sufferers? Was bone marrow transplantation the savior of sickle cell patients and their families, or was it a dangerous gamble, a high-stakes lottery in the world of medical innovation? Whether or not people buy the idea that we are on the verge of a breakthrough depends on the values they bring to such questions; it also hinges on whether they encounter health problems as patients and families, as medical practitioners, or as entrepreneurs.

As disorders of a genetic and ethnic "nature," these maladies have inspired intense and conflicted discussions over the decades. They have become subjects for high-profile legislation. In the 1970s the spotlight fell on sickle cell disease, on Tay-Sachs, and on such other diseases as thalassemia (a hereditary blood disease common among people from the Mediterranean—Greek, Italian, Israeli, and so on). As Congress pondered legislation to address these ethnic concerns, some suggested that this was simply "special treatment" for the newest "ethnic disease of the month." Within a few years, however, white Americans would have their own genetic disease to embrace: as if in response to the rising profile of these other maladies, cystic fibrosis came to be portrayed as "the white version of sickle cell disease."[11] Each disease, from time to time, has been an exemplar of both the best uses and the worst misuses of hereditary knowledge and genetic manipulation. They became potent sites for debates about family planning, religious values, and state intervention in the shaping of ethnic, racial, and communal identity. Not surprisingly, they also inspired fierce social controversy about the importance of autonomy and self-determination. In the shadow of these disorders, intense discussions would flare about the risks and benefits of innovative diagnosis and therapy and about whether genetics promoted or hindered the pursuit of social justice.

In the annals of medicine, these three diseases stand out as ethnic symbols for our time. As sociologist Herbert Gans noted in 1979, ethnicity was in transition in the late twentieth century. "Ethnicity may be turning into symbolic ethnicity," he said, "an ethnicity of last resort, which could, nevertheless, persist for generations." Gans observed that third- and fourth-generation ethnic immigrants in 1970s America had not erased their ethnic identity; nor, however, did they belong to ethnic neighborhoods, political organizations, or institutions, as had their predecessors. Their ethnicity was expressed more and more in symbols that had been given greater importance precisely because of the diversification and dispersion of formerly tightly knit communities. For example, Gans argued, once-minor rites of passage like the Bar Mitzvah acquired growing symbolic significance for Jews trying to maintain their ethnic and religious identity in the face of pressures for cultural assimilation.[12] Similar processes explain how Tay-Sachs disease acquired broader cultural significance as a Jewish disease problem in this era. The politics of symbolic ethnicity also inform discussions about sickle cell disease in relation to African-American identity and, on a subtler and often unrecognized level, shape medical and social ideas about the Caucasian disorder cystic fibrosis. With Gans's observations in mind, this book explores the ways in which therapeutic discussions that appear to be fundamentally about issues of biology and laboratory science are deeply enmeshed with questions of Jewish, white, and black identity in late-twentieth-century America.

Chapter by chapter, we move from Tay-Sachs disease to cystic fibrosis to sickle cell disease in a dialectical fashion. In chapter 1 the focus on TSD highlights the overarching role of Jewish identity politics and the struggle for Jewish self-preservation in shaping genetic medicine. In chapter 2, which focuses on CF, we describe the central role of therapeutic innovators and entrepreneurs in the story. Here, ethnic cultural issues play a far less obvious role. Yet as we shall see, white ethnicity—a symbolic amalgam of a wide range of historically diverse ethnicities—has been a powerful, if sometimes invisible, force in shaping public understandings of CF and genetic medicine. Then in chapter 3 we see how powerful ethnic dynamics combine with the drive toward therapeutic innovation in the history of SCD. This chapter describes the complex cultural entanglement of genetic medicine with the struggle for racial justice and fairness. We call attention to these themes because they arise out of the literature itself, and because they have played such defining roles in the histories of these disorders.

The conflicted and difficult history of genetics with regard to questions of race and ethnicity also casts its shadow in these accounts. In the early twentieth century, many hereditary scientists promoted the idea of the "inferiority" of black people and ethnic minorities. Tay-Sachs disease started its history with the label *Jewish amaurotic idiocy*. Following World War II and the Holocaust, and in the wake of the close links between eugenics and Nazi atrocities, geneticists distanced themselves from this eugenicist past and its notions of racial hierarchy and inferiority. The new genetics took a decidedly clinical turn, seeking to employ genetic knowledge not for social division and stereotyping but for improvements in the diagnosis and treatment of disease. Since its advent in the post–World War II years, genetic medicine has developed a more complicated relationship to questions of race and ethnicity.[13] As Diane Paul has argued, medical specialists who sought to eliminate disease genes had to demarcate their efforts sharply from past eugenic policies that targeted ethnic and religious minorities and the poor. Thus by 1968 one medical geneticist could say, "Eugenic goals are most likely to be attained under a name other than eugenics."[14]

The histories of Tay-Sachs disease, cystic fibrosis, and sickle cell disease reveal how the purported connections between disease and racial identity have been continually reworked to mesh with current politics, opinions, and social relations. At every turn, despite the biological impression of these categories, notions of "Jewishness," "whiteness," and "blackness" have thoroughly infiltrated the public and professional discussions about these maladies. Some biologists and social scientists assert, of course, that these are socially constructed terms rather than biological ones.[15] They stress that the long history of intermarriage and genetic exchange—between whites and blacks in America and between Jews of many regions and others—makes meaningless any claims about absolute genetic differences.[16] The same criticism holds for the category *white*, for it too is an amalgam of multiple regional, biological, and genetic identities from across the globe, evolving through complex patterns of intermarriage over time. Moreover, terms like *Jewish* that once connoted a profound biological and racial difference have changed their meaning in America. With intermarriage across groups, with a complex diaspora, and with a tendency to emphasize the cultural and religious meaning of *Jewishness*, biological notions have been pushed into the recesses of the historical past.

Race and ethnicity remain contentious topics in American cultural and political discourse, and the complexity and malleability of these terms have continued to confound us. Depending on where any commentator stands at any particular moment, Americans are capable of embracing any number of beliefs about race.

Some are comfortable referring to black people as a "race" despite long histories of cross-cultural contact and intermarriage and scientific arguments suggesting the meaninglessness of the concept. For others, *white* is a broad cultural category with powerful social resonance, even though white people might hail from many different regions and biological pasts. Some would insist, nevertheless, that *white* could indeed be understood as a biological label. The term *Caucasian*, even more than *white*, has been used to connote a biological identity along racial lines even though the term takes its actual meaning from a specific geographical reference — the people of the Caucasus region — that has bears little on American whiteness.[17] And what about Jewish Americans? In popular thought today, according to author Karen Brodkin (in stark contrast to one hundred years ago, for example), Jewish people are white. Yet Jewish people are often described in terms of ethnicity and religion (Orthodox, Conservative, Reform, secular). Adding to the complexity, terms like *Ashkenazic* and *Sephardic* introduce a biological element, pointing to the historical coherence of particular Jewish communities in Europe and Africa. The malleability, and the overlapping, of all these terms is striking. *Black* and *African American* (as well as the outmoded *colored*) also point not merely to changing conventions of naming people but to different boundaries around the group. Whereas *African American* stands in parallel to other ethnic identifiers, pointing to an African diaspora, *black* is at once more inclusive of all dark-skinned peoples and at the same time, in the American context, freighted with a history of derogation and insult as well as more recent connotations of pride and resistance. Despite the obvious fungibility of these terms, there remains a striking urge to treat these categories as timeless and concrete. This multiplicity of options — indeed, the very malleability of race as a category — has often swirled beneath the surface of discussions about Tay-Sachs disease, cystic fibrosis, and sickle cell disease. Our goal is to make visible the cultural meanings that, whether acknowledged or not, have attached themselves to these diseases.

Regardless of the historical and social complexities of race thinking, notions of biological blackness, whiteness, and Jewishness continue to have powerful cultural salience, and these three diseases operate as telling reminders of this assertion. For laypersons and professionals, for doctors and patients, for those who identify with these labels and those who don't, Tay-Sachs disease, cystic fibrosis, and sickle cell disease stand as powerful indices of the stubborn persistence of biological difference. Since their emergence into broader social discourse, they have served as symbolic vehicles for thinking about race and ethnicity in America. It is therefore no accident that these diseases should inform an ever-widening range of discussions: about therapy, about justice and fairness, about group identity, about the possibilities of genetic transformation, about the wisdom of screening and prevention, and about the promises and perils of innovation. What can Americans—whether black, white, Jewish, Asian, Latino, Native American, or other—expect from the genetics revolution? How do ideas about ethnicity become attached to disease and other symbols of suffering? This comparative historical study offers accounts of how these linkages are forged, and of how rich and often contradictory associations between race, ethnicity, and innovation flourish in the age of genetic medicine.

Although this book touches on many of the wrenching personal issues that emerge in the fight against disease, it should not be mistaken for an account of patients and families. Such an undertaking would involve detailed interviews, ethnographic study, and access to patient records over the decades as well as access to a broader range of personal narratives of illness than currently exists.[18] We base our analysis of these genetic disease histories almost entirely on published sources: written opinions, medical studies, and public commentary in various types of media. For us, the debates that appear in the pages of popular media like *Time* magazine and the *San Francisco Chronicle*, medical journals like *Blood* and the *New England Journal of Medicine*, and numerous other outlets, from *Discover* magazine to congressional hearings and law journals, provide powerful insight into the far-reaching cultural meanings of disease. The choice is deliberate, for we are fundamentally interested in the public face of these maladies and the ways in which this public record shapes the cultural meaning of disease. These sources reveal the constant play of group identity in the cultural, medical, and scientific imagination about these archetypal maladies. Of course, the way we tell this story is not entirely distinct from a patient's and family's perspective. For people with these disorders and their families, the issues of how other people have perceived their condition and portrayed it, how such actors have built investments in their experience, and how these interests have evolved over time must command significant attention, for these issues allow us to grasp more fully the plight of patients.

To be sure, in our society the fine-grained ideas and symbols that physicians and scientists generate in their clinics and laboratories communicate broadly and powerfully beyond those milieus. Using editorials, clinical studies, conference reports, and a wide range of popular media, we delve into questions about how writers have understood the therapeutic challenge, and into the cultural ideals of betterment, the remaking of bodies and selves, and social transformation. In these sources we discern popular ideas about how patients, families, and doctors define amelioration. Relief, we find, depends on issues such as the socioeconomics and nature of family life, the place of the family in their community and in the medical system, and the place of religion in people's lives. Ideas about therapy even depend on the politics of legislation and research funding and the vagaries of how the pharmaceutical industry develops products and markets the idea of better living through drugs.

In the early 1990s the genetics revolution seemed to be in its brilliant infancy, the promise of gene therapy shone brightly, and the puzzle of genetic disease seemed on the verge of being solved, at least in the thinking of many physicians and patients. In focusing our analysis in part on these years, we seek to pause and reflect on events that have moved with bewildering speed and momentum. The year 1993, for example, was one in which cystic fibrosis researcher Ronald Crystal confronted early setbacks in the effort to test CF gene therapy and sought to scale back on his earlier promises, insisting that "to think that we're going to have a cure . . . in a year is naïve." It was also the year in which *Time* magazine suggested that "a flavor enhancer may provide the first treatment for sickle cell anemia" because of its ability to "wake up genes." [19] Discoveries and claims came fast and furious in the early 1990s, and many commentators portrayed genetic disease as a solvable jigsaw puzzle in which the missing pieces were finally falling into place. Some observers feared, however, that technological progress was rapidly outpacing society's ability to sort out the good from the bad and to make informed ethical choices about how to use these new tools. With informed hindsight, we begin to see more clearly that genetic medicine was traveling not one path, but many. In this era, the stories of Tay-Sachs prevention, gene therapy for cystic fibrosis, and the perilous lottery for sickle cell patients suggested that the genetics revolution had brought these patients to three different crossroads, and that the promise of genetic manipulation of disease intersected with deeply held cultural views about risk and risk-taking. Each disease in its own way raised profound questions about how therapy was related to group identity and to the pursuit of social justice in America. In the pages that follow we seek to illuminate how these three apparently similar "ethnic" genetic maladies could have followed such different trajectories in the early 1990s, when the promise and peril of genetic medicine seemed clearly in view.

Diseases have powerful symbolic significance, both for the people identified with them and for society at large. One need only point to AIDS and its intersection with gay culture and politics, breast cancer as a women's disease, and prostate cancer as a male problem to get a sense of the profound relationship between disease symbolism and group identity. [20] In the case of a deadly infectious disease like AIDS, the symbolism became politically charged for those inside the circle of suffering in gay communities, and for those outside as well. With breast cancer, a particularly gendered body politics shaped the public meaning of the disease. And prostate cancer activists in recent years have attempted to build on these trends by linking a sense of male identity to what was once a little-known disease. As these examples suggest, disease symbolism serves many functions for insiders and outsiders, feeding into personal and community politics or playing a role on the larger social and political stage.

In the American context, genetic disease and genetic advances insert themselves squarely into the cultural politics and symbolism of family and community. In AIDS, breast cancer, and prostate cancer, as in Tay-Sachs, cystic fibrosis, and sickle cell disease, the politics of identity collides with biological theory, and the promise of genetic innovation becomes entangled with problems of justice, marketing, and hype. Families and entire communities, bound together by common ancestry, cultural heritage, and ethnic identity, are finding that they have high stakes in the rise of genetic medicine.[21] Innovations in the definition of disease often compel families to think of themselves differently, to rethink their relations with one another, and even to alter their behavior. Such a scenario was dramatized in the 1997 film *Twilight of the Golds*, about a woman carrying a fetus with a supposed "gay gene" and the family's intense conflict about whether to abort and what it would mean to bring such a child into the world. Although the film dwells purely in the realm of fiction, it draws our attention to the types of conflicts and dilemmas encountered and imagined by modern-day Americans, and it highlights the cultural narratives, the promises, and the pitfalls that have unfolded in recent decades around Tay-Sachs disease, cystic fibrosis, and sickle cell disease.

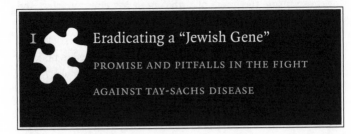

Since its discovery in the 1880s, Tay-Sachs disease (TSD) has always been experienced by parents as a tragic pathology, an inevitable downward spiral affecting very young children. One mother described the experience this way in the 1980s: At first her baby Ian appeared to be developing quite happily. He showed all the signs of normal infant development, only to begin missing a few developmental milestones. Motor skills he had gained early in life suddenly went into decline. Soon doctors diagnosed Ian with TSD, and his mother wrote, "Month 12 — cannot lift head when lying on abdomen; likes bath." The following months brought the child a wave of problems — an increasing loss of respiratory function, seizures, reduced interactions with the outside world, and life-threatening infections:

> Month 16 — mucus increasing — started postural drainage . . .
> month 17 — we bought suction machine . . . month 19 — started
> tube feeding . . . month 24 — seizes, vocalizes, grins, twitches
> (ironic that he looks so adorable, so "alive" during seizures);
> no other expression . . . month 25 — I think he hears . . . month
> 27 — has pneumonia — hospitalized eight days . . . month 29 —
> coughs well but not enough . . . month 31 — started antibiotic
> injections today . . . back in hospital for pneumonia; month
> 32 — home after 22 days . . . breathing very slow . . . feeding
> difficult.

Just short of Ian's third birthday, the sad and inevitable end came:

Month 33 — his lips do not move when we kiss him as they did last month . . . month 34 — stopped breathing during feeding on the 3rd . . . Ian was gone.[1]

Here was a powerful family drama, a narrative of relentless decline that would shape sensibilities not only about Tay-Sachs disease but also about ways to alleviate suffering in a wider range of genetic disorders.

Throughout much of the history of TSD (and still today), this course of decline for children with the disorder has remained unchanged. No breakthrough treatments or miracle cures could alter this inexorable decline, and until the 1970s, none were expected. Parents like Ian's mother hoped only for supportive care during the inevitable death of their child, and the intense experience of witnessing the decline of formerly healthy babies has overwhelmingly shaped how doctors and families think about therapy.[2]

The personal chronicle of the tragic deterioration and emotional burden of the Tay-Sachs child was a story that over the years became increasingly linked to the story of Jewish life and culture. The public history of Tay-Sachs disease has focused, therefore, not merely on generic parental suffering but on a particular kind of anguish: that of the Jewish parent. Because of the disease's historically high prevalence in Ashkenazic Jews, the medical conversation — about how to treat the child, how and whether to prevent such births, and how to eradicate such suffering — has taken on a particular cultural, ethical, and even religious significance. The symbolic connection between Tay-Sachs and Jewish people has made ethnicity and culture a prominent if not central concern shaping the promise of medical innovation.

Beginning in the late nineteenth century, a time of extensive migration for Eastern European Jews to new regions around the globe including North America, experts associated the disease with people they assumed to be a separate "race."[3] Characterized as "Jewish amaurotic idiocy" in the late nineteenth and early twentieth centuries, by the 1950s Tay-Sachs had been classified as a type of lipid storage disorder, a disease stemming from an abnormal buildup of fats in the body that can affect any one of numerous organ systems.[4] It was also often described as a lysosomal storage disorder, calling attention to the particular subcellular features of the storage pathology.[5] Other researchers have understood the disease in yet different scientific terms—as one of the "gangliosidoses" or the "cerebral sphingolipidoses," a framework that highlights the particular location of the lipid storage pathology in the neurons of the brain.[6] Each of these characterizations, starting with "Jewish amaurotic idiocy," has had important implications for how physicians, patients, researchers, and others have understood the core issues in the disease, and each has had important implications for framing possible approaches to therapy.

By the late 1960s and 1970s, scientific understanding had produced no effective treatment for Tay-Sachs disease, but advances had emerged in the realm of better diagnosis and prevention. In the absence of therapeutic gains, prevention had immediate and irresistible appeal for many of the Jewish families at risk for having babies with TSD. Beginning in the 1970s, American Jews embraced a wide range of newly available techniques to prevent the birth of Tay-Sachs babies. Among the novel methods used were mass genetic testing and reproductive counseling. If both members of a couple were found to be carriers, they might decide not to have children, or to take the chance—knowing the risks. Where prenatal genetic testing of fetuses was done, many American Jews chose to abort TSD fetuses. The results since the 1970s have been dramatic: the gradual decline of TSD among Jews living in the United States, and in many communities even its total eradication. In a relatively short time, TSD had been transformed into a modern genetic success story.[7] The number of family tragedies like Ian's was dramatically reduced.

As a strategy for disease prevention, the Jewish struggle against Tay-Sachs disease became exemplary, for it highlighted how modern genetics could support the value of ethnic self-determination in the modern era. Speaking in early 2003, one Stanford University population geneticist proclaimed that "Jews have taken charge of the information about diseases more common in Ashkenazis (i.e., Eastern European) and now accepted its usefulness."[8] Such comments drew attention to the fact that the success of this mode of disease prevention depended upon American Jews' embrace of the idea of genetic counseling, abortion, and other methods. They organized testing campaigns in colleges and religious institutions, encouraging unmarried people and potential marriage partners to find out if they carried the gene for TSD, and they warned couples who both carried the gene about the risk of conceiving a TSD baby (25% in each child). With some variations, Jews in Israel, Europe, and other parts of the world have also embraced this model. Thus, the decline of TSD among Jews in the 1970s, 1980s, and 1990s became an exemplar—until recently, at least—of the proper uses of genetic information in the name of self-preservation and communal health.

One of the major factors in the success of prevention has been the role of rabbis, religious leaders, and scientists in developing innovative techniques to spread information about the disease, and their role in shaping its meaning for diverse Jewish people. As suggested above, another motivating force has been the idea of Jewish self-preservation, which has played a compelling role for many Jews in shaping the practice of counseling, reproductive decision making, and making sure that fewer babies with TSD are born.[9] Of course, *Jewish* signifies not one but many different kinds of group identity. Increasingly the term *Jewish* evokes diverse religious communities and various cultural and secular practices. Some even argue that in recent decades American Jews have emerged as another "white" ethnic group.[10] Indeed, as efforts to bring TSD under control unfolded, this diversity in social conditions and identities among Jews was thrown into relief.

Diverse Jewish groups achieved dramatic successes in preventing the births of children with Tay-Sachs disease in an era when political and technological developments supported their efforts.[11] As one Orthodox rabbi put it recently, "Today, Tay-Sachs is almost non-existent in New York's orthodox community, and in Israel too. In the 1970s, the 16 bed Tay-Sachs ward in New York's Kingsbrook Jewish Medical Center was filled to capacity. Since 1996, the ward has had no Tay-Sachs patients." [12] As professional and media reports stated, genetic counselors, physicians, and rabbis worked together with family members in close-knit communities to avoid tragedy after tragedy. Political and social changes in the 1970s were also crucial to this success. Only then did selective abortion become increasingly feasible with the growing legalization of abortion. Amid frank pessimism about the possibilities of a cure, prevention of the disease by abortion was often characterized as "therapeutic." Indeed, the use of the term *therapeutic abortion* to describe the process reveals much about the era's liberalization of access to abortion and the shaping of such innovations by the cultural and social context of that time.[13] Even so, many Jews found therapeutic abortion to be an unacceptable means of TSD prevention.

Among some Jewish communities with strong religious proscriptions against abortion, these innovative methods could not be endorsed—and out of this tension the Dor Yeshorim was born. According to the Ultra-Orthodox view, abortion was just as tragic an outcome as Tay-Sachs itself. Other approaches would be needed, and this is why a new practice, the Dor Yeshorim, appeared in the 1980s. Dor Yeshorim (meaning "generation of the righteous" or "upright generation") initially emerged as a preferred strategy to combat TSD among some Ultra-Orthodox Jewish groups in New York and Chicago. It involved the testing of adolescent children within the religious community to determine whether they were carriers of the TSD gene. The practice was promoted as a new religious rite of passage, and adolescents found to be carriers would be restricted from marrying other carriers. Such restrictions ensured that the disease would never appear in their offspring. Rabbi Josef Ekstein of Brooklyn, New York, created Dor Yeshorim in 1983. Dor Yeshorim soon spread to other congregations in New York, in England, and in Israel, and it has since become a service available to high school and university students as well as a range of other young Jews judged to be marriageable. The fact that arranged marriage was already commonplace in many Orthodox communities made the innovation widely appealing, even logical.

The success of the Dor Yeshorim stood out, particularly in contrast with the toll that Tay-Sachs disease continued to take in a few other ethnic minority communities. In the early 1990s, just as the Dor Yeshorim emerged into a harsher spotlight, the upsurge in popular and professional awareness of Tay-Sachs also indicated that incidence of the disease was rising, not falling, in several non-Jewish communities, including French Canadians, Pennsylvania Dutch, and various Franco-American groups. In significant contrast with American Jews, the Franco-American religious community of New Hampshire was portrayed in media accounts not as a model for the local fight against genetic disease but as a persistent enclave of ignorance. One article noted, "Some researchers worry that a lack of information about the possible risk, plus ethnic pride and opposition to abortion, could keep New Hampshire's predominantly Catholic Franco-Americans from getting tested for the gene that causes the enzyme deficiency." [14] At the same time, the increased prevalence of the disorder in rural Louisiana fed into negative stereotypes about Cajuns. These were, of course, precisely the kinds of stereotypes about ethnicity and disease that some Ultra-Orthodox rabbis had encountered. In Louisiana, TSD became widely perceived as "the Cajun disease," a disorder that produced "lazy babies" and refocused attention on cultural stereotypes of Cajuns as "people who marry among themselves." [15] Such social portraits of Tay-Sachs in different parts of America — as part of the "bloodlines of the region" in Louisiana, as part of Catholic Franco-American culture in New Hampshire — highlight not only how the meaning assigned to the disease would depend upon the nature of community politics but also how the community's response could stigmatize the community itself. Against this backdrop, the Dor Yeshorim model of prevention would be hailed as a success. But clearly it would not find acceptance in many other locales.

By the early 1990s, the success story of the Dor Yeshorim took a dramatic, and some would say unfortunate, turn. As scientists produced more and more information about the genetic basis of many other diseases and about their prevalence in Jews, and as talk of more and more "Jewish genetic diseases" appeared in news accounts, it seemed prudent to incorporate new tests for genetic diseases into the Dor Yeshorim. Controversy quickly arose when Rabbi Ekstein and others advocated expanding the practice to test for and prevent marriage among carriers of genes for (among other disorders) cystic fibrosis and Gaucher's disease. Indeed, the inclusion of these two particular diseases drew attention to the fact that the Dor Yeshorim existed in a narrow ethical borderland, and that by spilling over from preventing a fatal "Jewish disease" to preventing other less deadly maladies, the program ran the risk of putting life with a chronic but manageable condition in the same category as life with Tay-Sachs. Since control rested firmly in the hands of the rabbi and families, geneticists could only complain, as did Michael Kaback, that the use of genetic screening to prevent manageable as opposed to fatal diseases threatened to transform what had once been seen as enlightened self-determination into an assault on self-determination and on genetic and human diversity. Kaback noted that the decision to target less deadly maladies created a problem: "Every single human being, you and me too, we have genetic risks for our children, whether it's cancer, early heart disease, or certain types of mental illness. I don't know where this stops, or who makes the decision where it stops."[16] The expansion of Dor Yeshorim thus raised a troubling question for many experts in the field. Was this expansion part of the dream of the new genetic era? Or was it, as Francis Collins, director of the National Human Genome Research Institute, would assert in 1993, a "nightmare"?[17]

What forces brought the fight against Tay-Sachs to such a perilous intersection in 1993? In many ways the story of TSD, the Dor Yeshorim, American Jews, and Gaucher's disease is a narrative of clashing values and perspectives in which ideals of genetic self-determination intertwined with deeply held religious values and notions of ethnicity and suffering. The story offers illuminating insights into the politics of ethnic community and into the promise and perils of community-based management of genetic information. It also reveals how the very meaning of *genetic disease* varies by community, place, and time, and how the notion of genetic disease is integrated into broader and historically bound senses of self, identity, and group. The debate over the Dor Yeshorim highlights an obvious but often unrecognized reality: that genetic diseases are not all the same, either in their natural course or in their cultural meanings.

Why does the concept of Tay-Sachs resonate with particular meaning for American Jews and to a lesser extent for those outside Jewish communities looking in? Only by considering the overall trajectory of TSD, as well as Gaucher's disease and (in a later chapter) cystic fibrosis, can we fully understand the tensions that surfaced over the Dor Yeshorim and its expansion, in the early 1990s, to other genetic diseases.

FROM "JEWISH IDIOCY" TO HEX-A DEFICIENCY

In the 1880s a British ophthalmologist (Warren Tay) and an American physician (Bernard Sachs) observed some of the crucial symptoms—the optical degeneration, the arrested cerebral development—that came to define Tay-Sachs disease.[18] The two physicians described how a child with Tay-Sachs, apparently normal at birth and into the first months of life, descended into severe retardation, early blindness, and epileptic seizures, followed by paralysis and death, often from pneumonia, usually by the age of three or four.[19] Little was said about the parents' perspective, but the clinical portrait was clear. Because of the slow degeneration, particularly of mental and optical (amaurotic) function, and its appearance multiple times in particular families, Sachs attached the label *amaurotic familial idiocy* to the disorder, and that descriptor persisted well into the twentieth century.[20] In the early stages of this drama of discovery, Sachs (a Jewish physician working among a large Jewish immigrant population in New York City) acknowledged that the disease was "almost exclusively observed among Hebrews."[21] However, he regarded it as a dispersed form of "familial idiocy," which was merely concentrated in, but not exclusive to, this new population of American Jews.

Scientific developments of the early twentieth century had no impact on the experience of Tay-Sachs disease; therapy offered little, but clinical understanding did advance steadily. Research on the disease in this era produced only an increasingly precise description of what was happening during the decline of infants and children with TSD. Through the 1930s, 1940s, and 1950s a more complex clinical and biological portrait of the disease emerged. By the early 1940s physicians could describe in detail why the infant slowly degenerated: it was apparently because of the excessive accumulation of specific types of lipids (fatty molecules called gangliosidoses) in particular brain cells.[22] They could do very little to remedy this accumulation or to stop the tragic decline. However, the very notion that they were dealing with a "brain disorder" — rather than, say, "amaurosis" or "idiocy" — opened up new lines of thinking about the distant, futuristic possibilities of therapeutic interventions.

New scientific knowledge provided clues about the linkage between Tay-Sachs and Jewish populations. For example, one important development at midcentury was the awareness that TSD was not a unique pathology but was part of a class of lipid storage disorders, and that this larger group was distributed across different populations. By the mid-1960s, researchers had isolated the subcellular lysosomal particles associated with the accumulation of lipids, and based on this development TSD could be conceived of as one among many lysosomal storage disorders.[23] Along with these descriptions of the underlying molecular characteristics of infantile TSD came increasing attempts to provide updated social profiles for these types of maladies. As a result, TSD's association specifically with Ashkenazic Jews—those descended from ancestors in Eastern France, Germany, and Eastern Europe—became a clear, specific, and powerful linkage. Sephardic Jews (from Spain and Portugal) and Mizrahim (from Northern Africa) did not experience high levels of this particular lipid storage disease. Researchers employed population studies to establish the relative prevalence of TSD in Ashkenazic Jews, a link first made in the early 1930s.[24] In subsequent decades and into the 1960s, biologists were breaking down the often monolithic category of *Jews* into different lineages, each with its own history, cultural practices, and disease risks.

Was Jewish identity a unitary racial and biological one? Clearly it was not. In the American context in the 1960s, to speak of Ashkenazic Jews, rather than Jews in general, was to draw attention to the particular subpopulation within a large, diversifying group of second- and third-generation American communities. These Americans were assimilating national cultural practices, moving to suburbs, giving up formerly intense attachments to the homeland, to clothing, and to traditional ways of speaking such as Yiddish. Yet they were also holding on to powerful notions of religious and cultural distinction. As they negotiated this tension, the motif of distinctive diseases and distinctive forms of suffering served to provide a powerful common reference point—what one might call a new form of symbolic ethnicity.

In the late 1960s came a dramatic diagnostic development that further refined medical and social thinking about Tay-Sachs disease and opened wide the pathway to prevention. TSD had lacked a high profile before then, and medical scientists had largely ignored it. As one researcher noted, TSD was "the last of the major [lipid storage disorders] for which the explicit nature of the metabolic abnormality remained unknown."[25] Knowledge about the precise nature of the abnormality in Tay-Sachs remained sketchy through the 1960s, whereas (by contrast) knowledge of underlying disease mechanisms in cystic fibrosis, sickle cell disease, and other genetic disorders had led to well-developed research agendas focusing on both therapeutics and diagnostics.[26]

A key discovery in 1969 turned the attention of patients and physicians back to the clinic and to potential treatments: Shintaro Okada and John O'Brien's identification of the enzyme responsible for the normal breakdown of lipids, which was missing in the child with Tay-Sachs disease.[27] Before then, the discovery that a child had TSD usually occurred only when the clinical manifestations appeared—when the neurological and cognitive decline, mental retardation, and cerebral seizures began, followed by loss of vision and motor control and death between the ages of two and six. The identification of the missing Hex-A enzyme made possible diagnosis of TSD infants before symptoms appeared and opened up the possibility that fetuses could be diagnosed in utero—and that abortion could save parents from the anguish of watching their apparently normal child degenerate and die.[28] This advance prepared the ground for a new image of the disease—one that Ashkenazic Jews and other afflicted populations could readily embrace.

As these diagnostic events unfolded, biologists were pondering why this gene and disease were concentrated in Ashkenazic Jewish populations around the world—and they generated many theories and speculations. Was this prevalence explained by patterns of Jewish intermarriage, they wondered, by the "ghettoization" and intermarriage of Jews in Europe, by the close-knit nature of such communities, or by some possible survival benefit to parents carrying the gene? The new image of Tay-Sachs disease that emerged in the 1960s connected new pathological understanding with notions of a historical Jewish identity. What historical and social mechanisms could account for the higher frequency of the gene causing TSD in Ashkenazic Jews than in Sephardic Jews?[29] Among the theories that emerged was the notion that the disease originated from a "bad gene" that had spread by intermarriage, by migration, and by patterns of reproduction among insular Eastern European Jewish communities. There was a great deal of wild speculation in this literature. One study of TSD, for example, suggested that the disease emerged at the end of the nineteenth century among Russian Jewish immigrants in places like New York City because "all these carriers were now concentrated in one small section of Manhattan Borough—the Lower East Side—which encompasses an area of about 25 city blocks . . . an even smaller geographical area than the Pale of Settlement" in Russia.[30] In some respects the gene was imagined to have its origins in the repressive social conditions of ghettos in Eastern Europe. Writing for *Discover* magazine in 1991, geographer Jared Diamond even speculated that the prevalence of Tay-Sachs among Jews is the result of a genetic "blessing" that protected TSD carriers (heterozygotes) against the tuberculosis that was endemic in the crowded conditions of the ghettos.[31] TSD therefore symbolized a history of a people's oppression. In the upsurge in such theories, the disease became a part of the mythos of American Judaism.

As these connections to the Jewish past emerged, new scientific studies simultaneously complicated the clinical picture and gave cause for therapeutic optimism. It was apparently not exclusively fatal, nor was it confined to infants. Diagnostic advancement in the 1960s and 1970s revealed that the standard portrait of lipid storage disorders needed revision, for it now seemed that such ailments ranged from the tragically severe (as in Tay-Sachs disease) to the unrecognizably mild. Moreover, once TSD was redefined as a Hex-A deficiency, researchers began to identify juveniles and adults with the deficiency who exhibited only *some* of the symptoms of classic Tay-Sachs. These other forms of Hex-A deficiency did not fit well with the traditional clinical or ethnic profile of TSD. Hex-A deficiency was not exclusively a lethal disease of infancy. "While infantile Tay-Sachs occurs more frequently in Ashkenazi Jews," noted one researcher, "the juvenile form of Tay-Sachs has no ethnic predilection."[32] This new subclass of delayed Hex-A deficiency was, however, usually fatal by the second decade of life. Thus, the development of the Hex-A model of TSD enlarged the definition of the disease, shifting the social profile slightly, and, most important, opened up the real possibility of further extending the life of the patient via enzyme replacement therapy.

In the 1970s, then, scientific and social developments seemed to be opening the doors simultaneously to prevention, therapy, and increased cultural awareness of the deadly disorder. A great deal had been learned about identifying would-be parents who had the potential to produce Tay-Sachs children and about identifying TSD in fetuses. A disease once regarded as a kind of feeble-mindedness had come to be understood as a brain disease, a lipid storage disease, and now a deficiency of the Hex-A enzyme. It had also become clear that TSD was just one of many such disorders, standing alongside Gaucher's in a growing array of lipid storage disorders. The ability to identify TSD carriers and fetuses, combined with broadened access to abortion, fostered the rise of a preventive approach to TSD. At the same time, a distant hope had appeared: that the identification of the missing enzyme in TSD might lead to a more effective therapeutic approach.

THE "FAILURE" OF ENZYME THERAPY AND THE TILT TOWARD PREVENTION

With the identification of the missing enzyme responsible for Tay-Sachs disease, hope ran high among parents and researchers that such knowledge would lead to an effective therapy. As Bonnie Friedman of the Health Services and Mental Health Administration (HSMHA) wrote in 1971, "With medical science already able to prevent certain inborn errors of metabolism and hopeful of correcting others, it may soon be possible to strike many disorders from man's list of neurological ailments." Throughout the 1970s researchers' attention would focus not on the disease's links to the Jewish past but on the possibility that enzyme replacement therapies would make it a manageable part of the Jewish future. Friedman concluded, "With detection and prevention of

Tay-Sachs Disease
"THE BEST-KNOWN JEWISH GENETIC DISORDER"

TSD, a rare inherited metabolic disorder, is associated with Jews of Eastern European (Ashkenazic) ancestry. The gene occurs more frequently among Ashkenazic Jews than other populations, according to decades-old studies. The incidence of TSD among Ashkenazic Jews has fallen dramatically in recent decades as a result of mass carrier screening. Much of the data on TSD has yet to be updated as the profile of the disease continues to change.

Carrier Frequency	1 in 25–30 Ashkenazic Jews
	1 in 29 French Canadians and Louisiana Cajuns
	1 in 200–300 general population (including Sephardic Jews)
Disease Incidence	1 in 2,500–3,000 Ashkenazic Jews (natural incidence)*
Inheritance	Autosomal recessive
Cause	Gene mutation on chromosome 15
Mechanism	Hex-A deficiency (also known as beta-hexosaminidase A deficiency). The deficiency prevents the body from breaking down naturally occurring fatty substances (GM2 gangliosides). These substances become toxic as they accumulate in the brain and nervous tissue and will progressively destroy the neurological system.
Symptoms	TSD is characterized by the onset of severe mental and developmental retardation during the first four to eight months of life. The child also develops seizures that are not controllable by drug therapy. After the second to third year the child is totally debilitated. Death typically results from pneumonia or another infection in the

	third to fifth year. (A late-onset form of TSD occurs in adults, but very rarely.)
Treatments	No effective treatment at this time
Screening	Carrier testing for adults can measure for Hex-A deficiency in the blood or use a genetic test to identify the TSD gene. Prenatal testing is possible using amniocentesis or chorionic villi sampling to identify whether a fetus has the Hex-A deficiency or the gene.
Prevention	Tay-Sachs screening programs, including the Dor Yeshorim, have detected tens of thousands of carriers in the last few decades, and many carrier couples in the United States have been counseled about their 25 percent chance of having a TSD baby.

*By most accounts, TSD among Ashkenazic Jews has fallen substantially from its "natural incidence." In 2003 and 2004, only ten TSD babies were born in the United States; none was Jewish.

Tay-Sachs disease possible, the question of a cure arises."[33] Within years, however, it became clear that TSD was not the best candidate for enzyme replacement therapy, and that there were several better candidates among the lipid storage disorders for this pioneering therapy.

Who might benefit from enzyme replacement therapy if not the tragic Tay-Sachs patient? Chief among the better targets for testing enzyme replacement therapy was the less well known lipid storage disorder Gaucher's disease, which came in several types. Type I was as prevalent among Ashkenazic Jews as Tay-Sachs, but its other forms were more widely distributed in the U.S. population.[34] Gaucher's (type I) was certainly not as symbolically power-

Tay-Sachs and the Dor Yeshorim

The Dor Yeshorim model for conducting TSD carrier testing among young Jewish people and encouraging them not to marry one another was created in New York City in the 1980s by Rabbi Josef Ekstein and then spread through other Orthodox Jewish communities. Considered a success by geneticists and community people alike, the practice generated controversy in the early 1990s when Ekstein decided to extend testing to several other, not invariably fatal, supposedly Jewish genetic diseases like cystic fibrosis and Gaucher's disease.

"I went knocking on the doors of community leaders, rabbis, anyone who was ready to listen to me and some of those who weren't, telling them that this was a problem and we had to do something about it. The point I made was that this was a problem for the entire community, not just for me . . . At the beginning of Dor Yeshorim, we had much opposition . . . But the idea caught on . . . and it gained support from other rabbis. Now testing has become part of Jewish culture."
—Rabbi Josef Ekstein, founder of the Dor Yeshorim, 2004

"As you move further and further away from an untreatable disease in which no one survives to cystic fibrosis and Gaucher's disease (in which the calculus of life, death and survival were starkly different), I find the application much more troubling and much less acceptable."
—Mark Siegler, ethicist, 1993

"When there is strong pressure within a community for members to have genetic tests and to check on the genetic profiles of whomever they date . . . this is a miniature but significant version of Big Brother . . . This is a moderate nightmare."
—Francis Collins, director of the National Human Genome
  Research Institute, 1993

"While ethicists agonize over some people's being marginalized as marriage partners, they would do better to focus on the fact that medical conditions not manifesting themselves until middle age

ful for Jews as TSD; since its discovery in the 1880s, Gaucher's had
never been associated with Jewish identity. Nor was it as dramatic
a disorder; it lacked the poignancy and personal tragedy of TSD.
Gaucher's was first designated as a lipid storage disorder in the
1920s.[35] But from the start, the Gaucher's experience was different
from the TSD phenomenon. Some of the types involved neurological complaints, as in TSD. But type I, the one that later was deemed
more prevalent in Ashkenazic Jews, was a much milder disease, involving none of the neurological symptoms characteristic of TSD.
Moreover, the disorder's onset during adulthood rather than infancy made it a dramatically different kind of family crisis. In comparison with TSD, discussion about either prevention or the possibility of enzyme replacement therapy for Gaucher's reflected a
very different set of experiences, histories, and cultural politics.

Why did researchers single out Gaucher's, not Tay-Sachs, as
a suitable candidate for testing the viability of enzyme therapy?
Roscoe Brady, a leading researcher in the field, noted in 1975, "We
are entering a new phase in the treatment of genetic diseases—
therapy by replacement of the deficient enzyme." This mode of
therapy, he speculated, "appears to offer much promise . . . for
patients with Fabry's disease and Gaucher's disease. However, en-

zyme replacement in patients with Tay-Sachs disease ... where the central nervous system is affected will require first the development of effective methods for the delivery of exogenous enzymes to the brain."[36] Researchers recognized that the neurological aspect of TSD—the involvement of the brain and the difficulties of getting drugs across the physiological blood-brain barrier—posed an almost unsurmountable obstacle to enzyme replacement therapy. By the late 1970s and early 1980s, however, clinical trials even on "best candidate" diseases like Gaucher's had produced ambiguous findings about the value of such agents.[37] Indeed, in 1977 Robert Desnick and James Goldberg would write that "unfortunately, the prospects for the treatment of Tay-Sachs disease are extremely discouraging."[38] In 1982 two noted researchers pronounced that "overall, the results of enzyme replacement therapy must be judged a failure" because of many factors: the failure to purify enzyme, the difficulty of delivering enzymes to the macrophage-monocyte system, the destruction of enzymes within the cells, and the poor capacity of enzyme to contact intracellular glycolipid deposits.[39]

The failure of enzyme replacement therapy in Gaucher's disease, researchers reasoned, meant that the therapy's prospects in Tay-Sachs were even worse. Enzyme replacement in the brain would have to involve passing macromolecules through the blood-brain barrier, and this was frequently cited as an overwhelming hurdle. Thus, even in this decade of rising expectations about enzyme replacement therapy, researchers uniformly affirmed that "because of the currently unsurmountable obstacles presented by disorders with primary neural pathology, research efforts towards enzyme therapy for lysosomal storage diseases have been directed to selected disorders without neural involvement."[40] Hopes for this mode of therapy would be raised again in the 1990s when enzyme replacement resurfaced as a promising treatment for Gaucher's disease. But in the 1970s and 1980s, when genetic screening and the Dor Yeshorim first emerged, there was little optimism regarding drug therapies for any of the lysosomal storage disorders. Prevention of Tay-Sachs thus seemed to be the best strategy for eradicating the disease, both for the present and quite likely for decades to come.

The promise of enzyme replacement was not extinguished entirely, however, and in later years the stories of Tay-Sachs disease and Gaucher's would follow different paths—one toward prevention, the other toward treatment. While the diagnostic advances and abortion policies of the 1970s had given rise to the prevention movement, the very different technological and legislative climate of the 1980s and 1990s pushed enzyme replacement back to center stage (at least for some diseases).[41] The passage of the national Orphan Disease Act of 1983 created powerful financial incentives for pharmaceutical companies to develop therapies for rare disorders (such as Gaucher's disease), research that would otherwise be financially unrewarding. In the wake of these legislative incentives, and amid the explosive growth of the biotechnology industry, enzyme replacement would make another appearance when the company Genzyme produced a new drug for Gaucher's. By the late 1990s, enzyme replacement was being hailed again as one of the important therapeutic promises of the era, standing alongside bone marrow transplantation for sickle cell disease and gene therapy for cystic fibrosis.[42] To be sure, the high cost of enzyme replacement and the pricing policies of Genzyme drew criticism.[43] But by the mid-1990s, enzyme replacement therapy for type I Gaucher's disease had gone from hoped-for remedy to dismal failure and back to clinical and market success. Hopes for those with lipid storage disorders again seemed warranted, and pharmaceutical companies nurtured these hopes in pursuit of profits. The promise did not extend to Tay-Sachs disease, however, for which few researchers or drug companies promised any therapeutic breakthroughs. While Gaucher's followed the new path of enzyme replacement, Tay-Sachs continued traveling the road of prevention.

The Dor Yeshorim emerged in the 1980s from scientific advances in diagnosis, and from a new politics of reproductive control. But its most important influence was the particular meaning of Tay-Sachs disease for American Jewish survival and self-determination. In the late 1960s the linkage between prevention and self-determination was highly politicized. There was, for example, intense public interest in the use of genetic counseling to prevent the birth of children with hereditary diseases, enabling parents to chart their own reproductive path and create healthy families.[44] The rise of amniocentesis, genetic screening, and reproductive counseling, coinciding with increased access to abortion, constituted a new approach to the prevention of hereditary disease. Politicians too saw this linkage as genetic counseling became a focus of national hearings and legislation throughout the 1970s, drawing public attention to the fight against a host of genetic diseases.[45] Prenatal screening and tests for a wide range of diseases promised to identify "otherwise healthy persons who possess genes that could be harmful to their offspring under certain conditions, and who could benefit from genetic counseling."[46] Autosomal recessive diseases like sickle cell disease, cystic fibrosis, and Tay-Sachs, in which the mechanisms and probabilities of inheritance were well established, attracted significant attention as candidates for eradication by means of the avoidance of birth.[47] Such discussions were, naturally, controversial; family or reproductive guidance offered by government officials in the name of public health threatened to impinge directly on considerations of religion, individual rights, self-determination, and the management of risks in diverse communities across the nation.

The very notion of managing a disease by controlling reproduction was fraught with risk for researchers and physicians, especially when their efforts seemed to target minority or disadvantaged populations. Genetic counseling for sickle cell disease, for example, had been highly controversial since its advent in 1972 and 1973, when it appeared to many African Americans that mandatory screening programs initiated by state governments were merely efforts to impose limits on the size of black families. For this community, genetic counseling quickly became associated not with empowerment but with efforts to limit the black population and with insinuations about black genetic inferiority. Issues like these were critical not only to black Americans but also to Jewish Americans, for whom the themes of population control, genetic inferiority, genocide, and community survival also had deep historical and religious resonance.

For Tay-Sachs and sickle cell disease, the prevention idea was tangled together with different questions of ethnic identity and minority survival in a majority White Anglo-Saxon Protestant America. To be sure, Tay-Sachs was a more uniformly fatal disorder than sickle cell disease, and for this and other reasons TSD took on tragic meaning for those concerned about the preservation of a strong and cohesive Jewish people. Much more than the suffering of children or the pain of parents was at stake here. Moreover, this concern was articulated by Jewish leaders themselves — not, as with screening for sickle cell disease, by politicians or government officials. It was rabbis and other religious leaders who brought up the issue of self-preservation and put themselves at the very center of the debate over how best to manage Tay-Sachs.

Because issues of cultural identity and survival were involved, researchers explored the possibilities of "preventive therapy" for Tay-Sachs disease with great caution and in partnership with community leaders. In doing so they showed that they had learned much from mistakes of the early 1970s regarding proposals for preventing sickle cell disease. The limitation of reproduction was a complex and controversial issue. Depending on how this goal was articulated, and who articulated it, the eradication of a gene could be seen as an act of self-preservation or an attempt at population control by unsavory outsiders. At least one author argued that "the Jewish community in America can be readily organized and educated through its various institutions to participate [in Tay-Sachs screening]" — implying that American Jews were culturally more accepting of professional or expert control than other ethnic groups.[48] At the same time, there was a strong aversion among some religious leaders to intermarriage — another effective method, of course, of preventing genetic disease. As one rabbi stated bluntly, "For a people which constitutes less than 3 per cent of the American population to countenance [high rates of intermarriage] is to jeopardize Jewish survival in the extreme."[49] Clearly any preventive therapy needed to address these social realities and political questions within affected communities. Who would control the flow of information about carriers? Who would weigh the possibilities of cure against the benefits of prevention? Who was in a position to evaluate the promise of research? Toward what ultimate end and for whose benefit would new information be used? And as this information was put to use, what would be the cost to individual self-determination? Each community would tackle these questions in its own way.

The particular features of the diseases in question added further complexity. Tay-Sachs, sickle cell, Gaucher's, and the others each had its own character, variability, burdens, and meanings. Despite the similarities in how "ethnic hereditary diseases" were passed from parents to offspring, there were crucial differences between the stories of Tay-Sachs and sickle cell disease, for example, as presented in popular, scientific, and political discussions. But most important, a huge gap in life expectancy and life chances confronted children born with these two disorders. Tay-Sachs disease presented the tragic scenario of a tiny child "cheated of the opportunity to live out his life," silently suffering a tragedy that could have been avoided if only the parents had received enough information through genetic screening and prenatal diagnosis to prevent its birth.[50] The child had no independent identity in public imagery apart from its suffering parents. There were no popular profiles of people living with TSD as there were for

sickle cell disease or cystic fibrosis. There were no dramatic portraits to match the Cystic Fibrosis Foundation's poster child and
no popular books comparable to Frank Deford's 1983 book *Alex*.[51]
The birth of a TSD baby was characterized as a tragic pathology
in itself. Avoidance of birth was the only hope. As one physician
said of TSD testing, "This test eliminates the possibility of pain
. . . you're saving a little life of interminable suffering. The whole
idea is to avoid that. Tay-Sachs, that's unrelenting pain and that
never goes away."[52]

Against this backdrop, the advent of new Tay-Sachs testing
technology and birth prevention transformed the emotional possibilities for parents and reshaped the ethical and legal landscape
as well. Prenatal testing was often assumed to be infallible. Indeed, some parents would pin their hopes on testing and prevention to such an extent that in cases where testing gave incor-
rect information and TSD babies were born, debate arose about
whether lab scientists and physicians could be held accountable
on the grounds of allowing a "wrongful life." Whereas an earlier
generation might have seen the birth of a TSD baby as fated, a new
cohort of parents might see such a birth as entirely preventable
and characterize errors in testing as "preventive malpractice."[53]

These disease prevention efforts took on particular meanings
for American Jews in the context of simmering anxiety about Jewish intermarriage and group survival in the 1970s and 1980s. The
post–World War II years had seen a mainstreaming of American
Jews into the larger culture. As historian Matthew Frye Jacobsen
has noted, whereas in "the latter half of the nineteenth century
Jews, by common consensus, did represent a distinct race . . .
by the mid-twentieth such certainties had evaporated."American
Jews "became white folks," in popular thinking, by moving to
the suburbs, losing accents, and integrating into middle-class life
and culture. But in the 1970s and 1980s attention shifted back to
themes of Jewish ethnic distinctiveness, group survival, and continuing coherence. The preservation of Jewish culture in families
became, according to one scholar, "perhaps the most striking fea-

ture of the Jewish family . . . each person filled with a sense of duty and responsibility toward the other."[54]

The theme of a people at risk resonated powerfully with the ideal of prevention that emerged in the 1970s. For many, screening, counseling, and selective abortion came to take on far-reaching "therapeutic" connotations.[55] Between 1971 and 1975, more than one hundred thousand Jewish people in America were screened for Tay-Sachs disease, producing information on carrier frequency in this population (later revealed to be 1 in 27.3 persons).[56] Screening was also encouraged by national initiatives like the National Sickle Cell Anemia, Cooley's Anemia, Tay-Sachs, and Genetic Diseases Act of 1976, which provided dollars for research, training, testing, counseling, and education for a wide range of genetic disorders.[57]

Even as screening programs detected more carriers and prevented diseases, controversy shadowed these efforts.[58] One of the pitfalls to genetic testing lay in how it was promoted. One physician, for example, objected to the promise of the Tay-Sachs prevention program that "detection and counseling [would] enable carrier couples to have children free of this disease." While on the surface the claim rang true, it was also misleading, he argued, because the ambiguous phrase "have children free of this disease" might be read by some people as a suggestion that "some therapeutic maneuver would somehow make the genetically defective child normal." Being tested and having offspring "free of the disease," he argued, needed to be more clearly defined as involving "amnioscentesic tests and then abortion."[59] The concern also arose that screening programs might stigmatize carriers of hereditary disease: "Modern [diagnostic] technology may have introduced a new biological and social label — 'carrier' — with yet unknown psychological and social consequences." How would families, communities, neighbors, employers, or insurers respond to the carriers of genetic disease? As two authors writing on the question of stigma noted, "We do not know what part an individual's religious affiliation or degree of commitment plays in his ability to accept his carrier status without denigrating his human worth."[60]

The pitfalls of testing and identifying carriers were numerous. The danger had become strikingly evident in the late 1960s when Linus Pauling suggested that a distinctive mark should be tattooed on the foreheads of children carrying the sickle cell trait so that they could recognize one another as carriers from an early age and avoid falling in love, marrying, and producing children.[61] Increasingly as well, the ethical pitfalls became more evident when screening programs began to preach about the economic benefits of testing and the social costs of genetic diseases. For some, heavy-handed persuasion of carriers to avoid pregnancy seemed warranted by the high financial costs to society, the "economic burden of genetic disease [being] substantial."[62] For others, however, such considerations went beyond the bounds of what a liberal society should encourage.

In this context, some authors wondered whether anxieties about genetic disease were being overplayed and oversold to Ashkenazic Jewish populations. What did it mean, they wondered, that the issue of Tay-Sachs disease in Jews had become suffused with religious and communal significance? Madeleine and Lenn Goodman noted with some consternation, "Brochures warning American Jews against genetic diseases are printed in blue on white, the colors of the Jewish prayer shawl and of the flag of Israel. One logo showed the profile of a child's face from which fell a single tear, inset into a Star of David."[63] The tear, they explained, referred to one method of TSD detection (teardrops were the fluid often tested).[64] But the emotional valence was obvious: this was a disease about which many tears had been shed in Jewish communities. Other scholars pointed out that the new trend toward genetic and reproductive counseling posed "special challenges" to Jewish people "because of the complexities of Jewish religious law" on matters of disease prevention and abortion, and "because of the collective memory of Nazi attempts at genetic control during the Holocaust."[65] Such commentaries acknowledged that discussions about Tay-Sachs would necessarily merge uneasily into larger discussions about Jewish genetic status, "Jewish genetic diseases," and the Jewish past, present, and future.

Thus, even as testing initiatives progressed from the 1970s into the 1990s, some physicians and ethicists raised questions about the detrimental effects of genetic screening, drawing attention to the perpetuation of noxious stereotypes about Jewish inbreeding and disease, the diversion of community resources that might be used in other ways, and the use of testing programs to increase the power of rabbis, religious officials, and community leaders. For other observers this was not a problem at all. Indeed, it seemed altogether good that such officials were involved. But according to Madeleine and Lenn Goodman, "Enlisting the aid of such leaders places them in the problematic position of advocating a preconceived ethical position to their constituents in the very circumstances in which the constituents might be turning to the rabbi as a source of independent guidance regarding ethically difficult choices." [66] Could it be that rabbis and other leaders were assuming inappropriate roles — taking on a fiduciary character with regard to their constituents? [67]

However controversial it was, the community-based battle against Tay-Sachs disease came to be regarded as an unqualified success. Jewish Americans' use of prevention as the best therapy was celebrated in the 1980s as an example of enlightened self-determination using new genetic information. The story seemed to represent one of the best examples of the meshing of genetic information with local values and the championing of self-determination by communities, individuals, couples, and religious leaders concerned with questions of morality and group preservation. For Tay-Sachs, the new age of genetic information meant that prenatal testing and abortion could prevent disease. The impact was far reaching. The example of Tay-Sachs prevention spawned new research questions about how and why different at-risk communities responded as they did to genetic risk and to this notion of disease prevention. It also established new expectations among would-be parents about genetic counseling and the birth process. Some observers began to ask whether physicians and counselors were keeping up with the fast flow of new information about Tay-Sachs disease and its at-risk populations.[68] Others began to ask whether after almost a decade of practice the TSD screening programs had accomplished their goals and at what cost to communities and families.[69] And despite the success of the prevention program, still others continued to ask if enzyme replacement therapy for TSD was ever going to materialize.[70]

The successful model of prevention via prenatal testing and abortion had definite limits as a cultural practice. For those with theological or political proscriptions against abortion, this mode of prevention was never an option. Orthodox Jews opposed abortion, and for some within this constituency the Dor Yeshorim represented an alternative path toward prevention and community health—a way to put the new genetic information to use without resort to abortion. For them, all that was needed were subtle adjustments to the rituals associated with adolescence. Indeed, as the Dor Yeshorim took shape and spread, it too showed that genetic testing could be integrated with specific moral and religious concerns. Identifying carriers, eradicating disease, and solving the Tay-Sachs problem need not include abortion, and could indeed support and strengthen the institution of arranged marriages among Orthodox Jews. This, to be sure, was a desirable "therapeutic" solution.[71]

Yet the community-based prevention of Tay-Sachs disease remained a positive model, particularly in an age of rapidly proliferating genetic information. Indeed, it was at this very time that "community consent" began to appear as a topic of interest in the medical ethics literature.[72] The story of TSD had several appealing features as a model. It involved a minority population as well as a minority within the minority group, both concerned with self-preservation and ethnic values. It also involved groups that were reputed to respect scientific information and that actively incorporated into innovative programs new information about their identity and risks of disease. In March 2003, noting that the Tay-Sachs unit in New York's Kingsbrook Jewish Medical Center now stood "completely empty," one professor of neurology asserted that it was "foolish, even criminal, for observant Jews not to undergo testing to prevent the birth of children with these dreaded diseases."[73]

Not all groups, however, waged similarly successful battles against Tay-Sachs disease in the 1980s and 1990s. French Canadians and Louisiana Cajuns, groups having very different identity politics, saw rates of TSD rise.[74] As in the case of American Jews, news accounts focused on issues such as inbreeding, group preservation, and the need to spread information about genetic status. The increasing incidence of Tay-Sachs in these non-Jewish populations would be seen as cautionary tales, however, and they only confirmed the exemplary nature of the TSD story in Jewish communities. However, when the architects of the Dor Yeshorim sought to expand the success of its "genetic matchmaking" service in the 1990s, the story line of success changed abruptly and a revealing clash emerged.

FROM DREAM TO NIGHTMARE? THE DOR YESHORIM

The religious and moral concerns that gave rise to the Dor Yeshorim were evident as early as a 1977 conference on Tay-Sachs disease, when tensions arose between Conservative and Orthodox rabbis. Each group worried about traditional Jewish law and its relation to the new issues of therapeutic abortion, to genetic counseling, and to the meaning of the life and death of the child with TSD. Noted one Conservative rabbi, "We recognize the trying ordeal which would be suffered by parents of a Tay-Sachs-diseased child . . . and therefore my own view is that the termination of pregnancy [via abortion] is morally defensible and halachically [i.e., in terms of Jewish law] acceptable." But for Josef Ekstein, the Ultra-Orthodox rabbi who had created the Dor Yeshorim, the problem was that prenatal screening had created a new set of problems. "A test was developed in the 1970s," Ekstein later noted, "but it was not used by the orthodox Jewish community because abortion is forbidden, so prenatal screening was out of the question."[75] For this rabbi, religious law could not sanction abortion as a means of avoiding the ordeal of Tay-Sachs even if it was understood as an intense form of familial suffering.

As agents of families in their communities, rabbis played a critical role in defining the moral and religious basis for this "therapeutics of prevention" into the 1980s and 1990s.[76] The distinct Jewish religious communities—Ultra-Orthodox, Orthodox, Reform, and Conservative—brought their diverse perspectives to the questions of family, community, and survival and to defining a meaningful approach to Tay-Sachs disease. In Orthodox and so-called Ultra-Orthodox communities, the Dor Yeshorim emerged as the sanctioned way toward TSD prevention.[77] Ekstein's original plan had been to carry out general premarital testing, but when other leading rabbis expressed concern about stigmatizing young people as carriers, a more circumscribed anonymous testing model emerged. Over the years, in practice this has meant that a representative of the Dor Yeshorim would distribute identification numbers to all individuals who one day might consider marriage. The individuals were then tested, either in religious schools or other settings, and whenever inquiries about potential mates would begin, the parties would exchange identification numbers and submit them to the Dor Yeshorim. The organization would quickly confirm whether the ID numbers indicated the genetic compatibility of the proposed couple. Ekstein used his influence to promote the practice while reshaping parental and community views about the disease. "A disease that runs in the family was a very taboo subject in our community," he later wrote. "Families who had children with diseases . . . didn't talk about it for fear that their healthy children would not be able to marry." The Dor Yeshorim changed this dynamic. "At first," Ekstein noted, "they didn't like it. Parents of sick children were afraid of their dirty laundry becoming public. The rest of the people did not know what I was talking about. But I knew that this disease was preventable, and the only way it could be prevented was if someone spoke out . . . I went knocking on the doors of community leaders, rabbis, anyone who was ready to listen to me . . . The point I made was that this was a problem for the entire community."[78]

The Dor Yeshorim, a kind of religiously sanctioned genetic matchmaking service, emerged out of a long series of discussions and fit neatly into Orthodox religious thinking about abortion, reproduction, religious hierarchy, and communal decision making. Noted one rabbi in 1990, "It is the obligation of every parent, without exception, to turn to Dor Yeshorim and heed their advice, before finalizing a match for his or her child."[79] Or as another authority noted more recently, people outside this tightly structured, traditional world "generally want autonomy over their bodies," but such notions carried less weight in Ultra-Orthodox culture.[80] The goal of the program was clear: "to eliminate Tay-Sachs from the Orthodox community, and to do it in accordance with strict Jewish law." For some Orthodox groups this meant eliminating the disease both without birth control and without abortions. As one author described the practice, "If a peek into a prospective couple's genetic code shows a bad match, they are discouraged from even dating and certainly from marrying."[81] The close ties of Orthodox communities, and parents' tight control over their children, ensured that such constraints could in fact be applied.

The Dor Yeshorim had a profoundly personal significance for Ekstein, who had witnessed the devastating effects of Tay-Sachs disease in his own family. By 1983, when he started the practice, his wife had given "birth to four Tay-Sachs children one after another, all of whom died before the age of six, even though the risk of the disease in children born to two carriers is 25% for each pregnancy."[82] Within a decade of the creation of the practice, Ekstein could note proudly that "8,000 young people were tested each year for the recessive genes." The Dor Yeshorim rapidly spread to other Orthodox communities in California, Tennessee, Michigan, Florida, and other states, becoming something of an "adolescent rite of passage."[83] As of 1993, sixty-seven New York couples who had been considering marriage had decided against it because of the risk.[84]

But controversy flared in that same year when the Dor Yeshorim in New York sought to expand to include testing for diseases that were not as severe as Tay-Sachs but that had become widely linked to so-called Jewish genes. In many respects, this was an understandable effort to build on a successful program by using new developments suggesting a linkage between other diseases and Jews. As one newspaper described the practice:

> Every year, Dor Yeshorim representatives go to the private high schools where many Orthodox families send their children and explain to the teen-agers that they can have a simple blood test to see if they carry genes for any of three diseases, Tay-Sachs, cystic fibrosis and Gaucher's disease. [Cystic fibrosis and Gaucher's were the new diseases to be tested that had shown a higher incidence among Jews.] Those tested are given a six-digit identification number. If a boy and girl want to date, or if they have already started dating, they are encouraged to call the New York Dor Yeshorim Central Office Hotline with their identification numbers. Then they are told either that the match is compatible — that they are not at risk of having children with the diseases in question — or that they each carry a recessive gene that could result in a child with one of the diseases.[85]

This expansion of the Dor Yeshorim program, though modest, raised serious questions for those outside the boundaries of Orthodox Jewish communities.

Experts ranging from medical ethicists to the head of the National Human Genome Research Institute denounced the expansion of Dor Yeshorim testing, calling it ethically and morally troubling. It was one thing, they insisted, to prevent the birth of babies with the deadly disease of Tay-Sachs, but quite another issue to extend the practice of "genetic matchmaking" and birth prevention to manageable disorders like cystic fibrosis and Gaucher's

disease. Ethicist Mark Siegler put it this way: "As you move further and further away from an untreatable disease in which no
one survives to cystic fibrosis and Gaucher's disease (in which
the calculus of life, death and survival were starkly different), I
find the application much more troubling and much less acceptable." Francis Collins, director of the National Human Genome
Research Institute, allowed that some aspects of the Dor Yeshorim
programs "sound just fine." Misgivings emerge, however, "when
there is strong pressure within a community for members to have
genetic tests and to check on the genetic profiles of whomever
they date." Such experts feared the prospect of coercion. They
also objected to the idea of preventing the birth of babies who
had diseases for which there were (or promised to be) effective
treatments, or who carried genes for diseases that might be mild
or that might manifest themselves only much later in life. Where
would this practice lead, they protested? Collins noted conclu-
sively, "This is a miniature but significant version of Big Brother
. . . This is a moderate nightmare."[86]

Control over these practices continued to rest, however, with
the community, not with outside experts, and a few days after the
publication of the newspaper story describing the expanded testing program, one observer shot back at the ethicists and geneticists: "While ethicists agonize over some people's being marginalized as marriage partners, they would do better to focus on the fact
that medical conditions not manifesting themselves until middle
age [like Gaucher's disease and cystic fibrosis] do not make them
benign or pleasant to live with . . . Prevention beats remedy any
day."[87] Other screening programs in nearby New York medical
schools were also exploring the idea of introducing screening
for cystic fibrosis and Gaucher's disease in conjunction with Tay-
Sachs carrier screening.[88]

Expert criticism of the Dor Yeshorim seemed, in the short term,
to have little impact on the practice of screening for more genes in
order to create healthy matches. The extension of the practice was
seen as a victory, a "pioneering scheme" in the eradication of dis-

eases. But the Dor Yeshorim in its new incarnation was no longer an unambiguous exemplar, a model of genetic disease prevention. The criticism, noted one commentator, had put Rabbi Ekstein "on the defensive against geneticists worried by the programme's extension to two other inherited diseases." In cystic fibrosis, for example, the troubling reality was that the Dor Yeshorim was preventing the birth of people who could live into their fifties.[89]

What factors drove the expansion of the Dor Yeshorim? The awareness that we all have genetic risks had been growing quickly throughout the 1980s and 1990s as genetic studies churned out more and more information about the links between genes and diseases. In some respects it was this very flood of new information about disease genes and their prevalence in the population that provoked the expansion of the Dor Yeshorim. As new information came along, the key question for doctors, patients, policy makers, and society at large was whether to expand the genetic testing services offered. Many rabbis had become closely tied to the world of genetic scientists, and extensive screening in Tay-Sachs had made a generation of Ashkenazic Jews more available to medical genetics research—research on not only Tay-Sachs but a range of other disorders—than at any time in the past. The result of this cooperation had been an explosion of knowledge and theories about a range of so-called Jewish genetic diseases.[90]

By the mid-1990s, scientists were openly speculating about the links between cancer, genes, and Jewish identity, thus raising the stakes for the Dor Yeshorim.[91] The new information raised the question of when testing should be done and when it should be curtailed. Rabbi Ekstein himself, the founder of the Dor Yeshorim, noted that he "would never test for genetic diseases that have dominant genes (which increase the risk of cancer, for example)." Amid the reports of two genes (BRCA1 and BRCA2) linked to a high risk for breast cancer in Jewish women, Ekstein commented that these genes were very different from genes for Tay-Sachs: "Knowing [that one carried the BRCA1 gene and could pass it on to one's children] could cause a patient much harm when making life decisions." Not only were the inheritance patterns of these genes not as straightforward as in TSD, but also such testing fit less neatly into the moral world of Orthodox Judaism: "Knowing they carry defective genes can cause low self-image, so we are determined not to test for defective dominant genes." In addition, the BRCA1 gene did not carry the same inevitable consequences of death associated with Tay-Sachs. Ekstein noted that for women with BRCA1, cancer "was not inevitable, unlike children born with two harmful recessive genes."[92] Ekstein's conclusion was clear: there would be no testing in the Dor Yeshorim for breast cancer genes regardless of their prevalence among Jewish women.

The discoveries of such disease-causing genes during the 1990s, however, created an increasing pressure to test. Studies proliferated, purporting to have found the gene for one thing or another: homosexuality, obesity, breast cancer, deafness, and many, many more. Americans began wondering which of these assertions were speculative, which were merely suggestive, and which were real causes for concern. In November 1998, for example, a *New York Times* headlines blared, "Gene Identified as Major Cause of Deafness in Ashkenazi Jews." As if to clarify the ambiguity of the headline, the text noted that the discovery did not mean that there was more deafness among Jews than in other groups. It meant only that scientists believed they had found "a particular genetic mutation that is more common among deaf Jewish people than among deaf people from other backgrounds."[93] Despite the many caveats attached to these findings, shortly afterward the Dor Yeshorim in New York began receiving requests for testing from families in which deafness had occurred, which compelled Ekstein to state that he was not sure that this service would be provided.

The logic of the marketplace and the possibility of profiting from diagnostic testing also exerted pressure on programs like the Dor Yeshorim. By the 1990s, nearly ten years after its creation, the Dor Yeshorim was no longer merely a benevolent nonprofit institution but a large money-making venture. With the cost of a test hovering around $250, one Ultra-Orthodox rabbi argued that genetic testing had become "a multi-million dollar industry" that was aggravating anxieties about inherited diseases and stirring up irrational fears about "so-called bad genes among people with little knowledge of human genetics, and that includes rabbis."[94] As one team of New York researchers noted, "New tests can be readily incorporated into established heterozygote screening programs." Moreover, the successes in screening for Tay-Sachs disease had created an atmosphere favorable toward testing: "The Ashkenazi Jewish population . . . tends to choose testing for all conditions for which heterozygote screening is available."[95] By 2005, according to one estimate, eighteen thousand people were tested annually by the Dor Yeshorim.[96]

This pattern of expansively testing Jewish bodies created its own new dilemmas. By the 1980s and 1990s the Ashkenazic Jewish population had come to provide a large body of data for use in a growing number of genetic tests and studies. Tay-Sachs screening programs brought thousands into clinics, where their blood samples could be tested not only for that disease but also, increasingly, for other genetic abnormalities. New information about genetic diseases in this study population emerged, and with it came the unfortunate tendency to suggest that these new problems were also "Jewish diseases" without having done studies in other populations. Publicity about such studies suggested, in turn, a uniquely tainted population, even though their authors struggled to make clear that their findings did not mean, for example, that deafness was especially prevalent among Jews or that it was any more due to genetics in Jews than in other groups. The research merely indicated that a gene had been found in this group; and the possibility existed that the same gene or similar ones would be found in other groups. Studies sometimes pointed out that because this group had made itself available for testing, it merely happened to be the group discussed. But such details were often buried far beneath the headlines; such distinctions were often blurred in media reports on "Jewish genes" and "Jewish diseases." By the 1990s, then, it had become quite clear to Rabbi Ekstein and others that there were both new promises and new dangers in becoming a target population for screening in an age of ever-expanding genetic information and services.

Not surprisingly, tensions emerged within the community over the implications of the increasing scientific and public focus on Jewish diseases.[97] Even as some urged the widening of disease testing, rabbis like Moshe Tendler worried that the focus on Jewish genetic diseases threatened the repetition of an awful past. In November 1999, as reports of other Jewish genetic mutations and disease appeared in the news and as the Dor Yeshorim was reconsidering whether to expand its services, Tendler worried "about possible discrimination from employers who might hesitate to hire someone prone to a genetic disease." At the time, amid national outrage over the practice of health insurance companies "cherry-picking" healthy policyholders and denying coverage to people at high risk for disease, concerns about genetic discrimination reflected anxieties about both ethnic discrimination and discrimination based on health status. Such talk about Jewish diseases sent a message that actually threatened Jews and that "could encourage anti-Semites who believe, as Adolf Hitler did, that Jews have 'bad genes.'"[98]

By 2000, acknowledging a wide array of concerns, the Dor Yeshorim had removed Gaucher's disease from its list of targeted diseases. Although parents were given an option to test for Gaucher's, mandated tests now included only Tay-Sachs, Canavan's disease, cystic fibrosis, and Fanconi's anemia.[99] The decision is revealing, for it highlights the facts that Gaucher's disease had acquired a very different meaning by 2000, that there was significant disagreement about the wisdom of preventing some diseases, and that the biotechnology and pharmaceutical industries' great hopes for treatment were inconsistent with the ideology of prevention.

What constitutes success in the management of heredity and disease? Who determines what is and is not a success? Such questions highlight that, in a diverse and liberal society, the dream of disease control will often be contested. The rise of the genetic matchmakers must be seen as one part of the continuing search for minority group self-determination through enlightened self-management. But by the 1990s the story of Tay-Sachs disease had unearthed deep-seated concerns about how and whether this prevention model should be extended. Some observers speculated that if the prevention approach worked for TSD, it should also be tried in Gaucher's, cystic fibrosis, and other genetic disorders. Yet the social logic of prevention was not the same in all diseases or in all groups. The success or failure of the new genetic medicine—whether genetic testing, gene therapy, or tailored drugs (pharmacogenomics)—can never be separated from practices of self-management and disease prevention in families and communities. Indeed, the effort in the 1980s and 1990s to expand the TSD prevention model to a wider spectrum of lipid storage disorders made clear the enormous differences among so-called genetic diseases, the multiplicity of views about eradicating such diseases, and even the variations within each disease and community. What once appeared to be a model example of how a small ethnic/religious community could be organized to eradicate a deadly disease evolved in 1993 into a complex, controversial case highlighting the pitfalls of social engineering.

PREVENTION VERSUS CURE: CONFLICTING GENETIC WORLDVIEWS

The controversy over testing for Gaucher's disease reflected a clash of values, a tension between two cultural perspectives, both rooted in powerful and arguably successful ideologies. One ideology focused on ethnic group preservation by means of prevention, the other on imminent cures and the role of the marketplace in bringing them about. Tay-Sachs was closely associated with the former ideology, Gaucher's with the latter.

Gaucher's disease and Tay-Sachs provide a striking example of how two genetic maladies can border one another and yet take on profoundly different cultural meanings and travel different historical paths. With Gaucher's, these meanings were shaped not so much by the politics of ethnic self-preservation, or even by its association with a particular ethnic group, as by other political and economic forces. Despite Rabbi Ekstein's view that it was one of the many genetic diseases threatening the Jewish population, Gaucher's disease had followed a very different historical trajectory from Tay-Sachs and by the 1990s had become closely associated with the a burgeoning biotechnology enterprise and its promises of impending breakthroughs.[100] Moreover, Gaucher's did not call to mind the powerful image of inevitable decline that haunted would-be parents and shaped public and medical discussions about Tay-Sachs. The ideals of community-based prevention that had worked so well with Tay-Sachs could not be easily applied to the eradication of Gaucher's, nor could screening "successes" be easily translated from the one disease to the other.[101] Indeed, the pharmaceutical management of Gaucher's offered a contrasting model of success, one that embraced but also transcended the disease's categorization as a "Jewish" malady.

Although Tay-Sachs disease and Gaucher's are considered to be in the same family of lysosomal disorders, the differences between them are extensive. Perhaps the most striking difference is that Gaucher's, discovered in 1882, comprises such a diverse range of clinical phenomena. The disorder causes erosion of bone tissue and fractures and can be characterized by episodic bruising and bleeding.[102] But in many people with Gaucher's, these symptoms may never rise to the level of a complaint. The symptoms range from nonexistent to mild to severe, and onset can come at any time—in infancy, adolescence, the middle years, or old age. Another difference, perhaps a crucial one from the standpoint of testing, emerged only after the 1980s: among those with the gene for Gaucher's disease, only 30 percent will ever manifest the disease. By the 1990s it was known that seven out of every ten people with the gene for Gaucher's disease would never show signs of illness or experience anything other than normal longevity and health. The screening of parents or fetuses for Gaucher's thus raised profound questions about just what was being prevented and what risks were being managed—especially since the disease was in no sense inevitable for those carrying the gene.

Issues of Jewish identity had never been historically central to Gaucher's disease as they had for Tay-Sachs. Its public profile in the 1990s was not as a Jewish genetic disease but as an "orphan disease": a disorder whose rarity made it—in stark contrast, for example, to cancer or heart disease—an unlikely target for pharmaceutical research, the numbers of patients being too small and the potential for profit too slim to make research financially attractive. Passage of the national Orphan Disease Act of 1983 had drawn attention to such diseases, giving drug companies a range of financial incentives to conduct research on these maladies and to develop drugs for them.[103] This legislation—enacted in the Reagan-era climate of deregulation, supply-side economics, and federal incentives for economic innovation—raised the political and economic profile of Gaucher's disease. Companies such as the Boston-based Genzyme came to recognize the potential for profit in genetic treatments for Gaucher's and other such diseases. By the end of the 1990s, enzyme replacement for Gaucher's had become a profitable enterprise and an option, albeit an expensive one, for many patients.[104] This scientific, therapeutic, and marketplace success stood in marked contrast to the story of Tay-Sachs disease and helped push the older model of preventive management toward the margins of the fight against genetic disease.

Was the Dor Yeshorim's program of Tay-Sachs screening and prevention a model for other diseases? Or were new trends in therapeutic innovation and pharmaceutical investment pushing prevention to the margins? In 1993, those who opposed the inclusion of Gaucher's in the Dor Yeshorim program, medical geneticist Michael Kaback among them, believed that disease testing had been oversold to the public. Scientists had oversimplified the benefits of genetic screening with the message that "if a test exists, you should use it." This mentality obscured the manifest differences between various genetic disorders. When TSD strikes, Kaback noted, it is always fatal and demoralizing for all concerned. By contrast, only a "minority of people [with Gaucher's] have severe and painful symptoms appearing in childhood . . . The first symptom usually does not surface until about age 45 [and] many people never know they have the disease." Accordingly, Kaback cautioned against extending the Dor Yeshorim's genetic screening efforts from Tay-Sachs to Gaucher's. Tay-Sachs, he argued, was the exception among genetic diseases, not the rule, and so "when they start packaging other things in there [with Tay-Sachs], I get real concerned."[105]

By the late 1980s it also seemed clear that an effective enzyme replacement therapy for Gaucher's was on the way, and on 5 April 1991 the FDA approved macrophage-targeted glucocerebrosidase as a specific treatment for the disease.[106] The financial incentives built in to the Orphan Disease Act also now came into play, turning Gaucher's into a more attractive subject of research for drug companies. Genzyme, a leading player in the growing biotechnology industry, used the enzyme replacement research of Roscoe Brady at the National Institutes of Health to move into the business of Gaucher's disease management.[107] By 2000 Genzyme was the second-largest biotechnology company in New England, with 75 percent of its 1999 revenue coming from its Gaucher's drugs Cerezyme and Ceredase (Cerezyme's predecessor).[108]

While the expense of enzyme replacement was prohibitive for many patients, estimated at $100,000 per year in 1993, Kaback and others suggested that avoiding that high cost was not a sufficient reason for parents to abort or prevent a Gaucher's baby. Avoiding the pain of infant death from Tay-Sachs was one thing; avoiding the high cost of care for Gaucher's was quite another. Even Ekstein agreed. In 1993, when the Dor Yeshorim extended couples testing to include Gaucher's, he observed that "with Tay-Sachs, there may be ethical reasons to abort . . . But there is no ethical reason to abort a Gaucher's baby."[109] While the remark would seem to reopen the door to abortion for Orthodox Jews seeking to avoid TSD, it also reveals Ekstein's awareness that the growing ability to treat Gaucher's made the extension of Dor Yeshorim screening a matter of controversy in the American Jewish community. This was not merely an ethical conundrum but a dilemma born of the different historical trajectories of the two diseases. The way in which Gaucher's had been pushed into the public spotlight as an orphan disease had given it a powerful cultural label that distinguished it quite clearly from Tay-Sachs, which had evolved in public thinking as a tragic inheritance among Ashkenazic Jews.

Many observers in American Jewish communities—as well as in Israel, where Gaucher's disease was likewise a prominent concern and where its treatment was covered under the national health plan—saw compelling parallels between Tay-Sachs disease and Gaucher's. After all, the prevalence of type I Gaucher's was higher among Ashkenazic Jews than among any other population. Who, then, was to say whether the disease was a "Jewish disease" or not? Who was to say what level of disease and distress should be singled out for prevention? And in the wake of therapeutic success, what kinds of commitments should be made to get expensive treatments into the hands of patients?[110] While almost no one quibbled over the wisdom of preventing TSD births, prevention of Gaucher's raised hackles in some quarters. For most observers, Gaucher's did not speak to questions of Jewish survival, self-preservation, and identity but rather highlighted a different set of cultural questions: How could government incentives, pharmaceutical innovation, and a fair marketplace for drugs help people confront this rare, variable, but treatable disease? Who would pay for the expensive drugs? And how would society at large respond to the needs and burdens represented by individuals with the disease?

To place Gaucher's in the context of the American political economy is to understand how constituencies very different from those in the TSD story shaped the lives of individuals affected by the disease. An array of historical forces came to bear on the question of whether prevention constituted success. In the case of Gaucher's disease, the growing national commitment to biotechnology changed the very meaning of *success* and *failure*. Biotechnology breakthroughs convinced some observers that Gaucher's and cystic fibrosis were radically different from Tay-Sachs disease and that the Dor Yeshorim expansion was truly a "moderate nightmare." But in 2004, Rabbi Ekstein remained proud of the fact that the Gaucher's test was still offered: "We now test for nine different diseases, with the option of testing for Gaucher's disease, a condition that is not always severe and one that can be treated, but only at great expense." For Ekstein, the high price of drug therapy and the greed of pharmaceutical companies were sufficient reason to keep offering the test.[111]

A crucial difference between the two diseases was this: Although Gaucher's disease (type I) had been recently integrated into a Jewish sense of group identity, it was not freighted with the same meanings as Tay-Sachs. It did not connote the threat of the Jewish people's disappearance or a legacy of suffering and pain. For Ekstein, the tension over whether to prevent births of Gaucher's babies highlighted a clash between business and community perspectives. For him, any limits on a group's power to manage its gene pool and to shape its genetic destiny should be determined by the ethos and values of the group itself.

THE PERILS OF GENETIC MATCHMAKING

By the early 1990s, the prevention of Tay-Sachs disease in Jewish communities stood as an exemplar of the success of community-based prevention programs in general. As such, it is quite understandable that the architects of the Dor Yeshorim would seek to build on the prevention model that had helped to reduce rates of the fatal disease. But this image of community control shifted in the 1990s, and what had been regarded as a model program also came to symbolize the misuse of genetic information.

The expansion of genetic disease prevention programs proved

controversial for various reasons, among them the fact that new knowledge was constantly reshaping the meaning and the symbolism of all diseases. In the age of genetic medicine, with new information constantly becoming available about a widening range of obscure genetic conditions, TSD evolved from an archetype — the prime example of a preventable genetic disease for which testing was desirable — into an anomalous disease so lethal and tragic that it no longer stood as an appropriate model for the prevention of other genetic maladies. To understand the controversies regarding the Dor Yeshorim, then, we must look to these changing meanings and contexts: to developments in the identification of nonfatal, chronic genetic diseases, to cultural ideas about the meaning of these disorders in various communities, and to a shift in focus to groups other than the Ultra-Orthodox Jewish communities that had created and embraced the Dor Yeshorim.

A wide array of actors and forces shaped the success or failure of genetic disease prevention efforts. The imperatives of prevention ("if you have a test, use it") continued to appeal to patients and practitioners alike. Michael Kaback noted that "this mentality, unfortunately, has been fostered in some degree by the scientific community." [112] To be sure, disease testing was also a money-making enterprise (as was drug development). But in the end, scientific developments, economic interests, religious ideals, and the social dynamics of family and community life combined to alter the path traveled by each genetic illness. [113] Gaucher's disease might resemble Tay-Sachs in some ways, but in the broader cultural context they are profoundly different kinds of pathology traversing different pathways.

In the cultural terms of the day, the movement to eradicate TSD in the 1970s and 1980s was a success story — one that stood in stark contrast to other prevention efforts. It was an exemplary case of genetic information positively applied to the eradication of disease, an affirmation that scientific intervention can be carried out in a way that respects community values and cultural self-determination. To this day it is often contrasted with the more angry and contentious story of sickle cell disease testing in the 1970s (discussed in chap. 3), which many in the black community saw as an attempt to coerce black families into having fewer children. In both black and Jewish communities, success and failure in the fight against genetic disease hinged on crucial differences in how communities perceived the risks and promises of testing, how society portrayed the disorders, how experts made their cases for treatment or prevention, and how communities responded to new scientific knowledge.

The story of the Dor Yeshorim makes abundantly clear how ideas about the proper uses of genetic information changed dramatically between the 1970s and the 1990s as society itself changed, as scientific discoveries proliferated, as questions regarding the role of governments arose, as crises of ethnic identity emerged, and as the understanding of disease mechanisms evolved. Far more than ethnic group identity was at work in shaping the story of Tay-Sachs disease. A wide range of other factors — scientists and their ideals, the interests of particular communities, the specific characteristics of the disease experience — accounted for its trajectory over time.

In the end, Tay-Sachs disease and Gaucher's were superficially similar and yet profoundly different, not only as experienced by patients and in their biology but also in their demographics, in their histories, and (perhaps most important) in their political, economic, and cultural meanings. Despite their kinship as genetic diseases, they raised profoundly different questions about risk, therapeutic choice, and group identity. Moreover, their contrasting trajectories affirm that the promise of scientific innovation has had radically different implications for the management of different genetic disorders over the decades. From the discovery of lipid storage disorders and new understandings of Hex-A deficiencies, to the rise, fall, and resurgence of enzyme replacement therapy, to the advent of the biotechnology industry, the paths of TSD and Gaucher's also illustrate that the very terms we use to characterize these disorders (e.g., the phrase *genetic disease*) convey very little about the diverse viewpoints, cultural complexities, and group notions of suffering represented by disease.

Can familiar truisms about race biology, ethnicity, or culture capture the complexity of the story of Tay-Sachs disease? The issues revolving around the management of the disease go well beyond racial or cultural concerns, for the story raises fundamental questions about community, identity, and the dream of genetic medicine. How do groups associated with certain diseases see themselves in the world? How do they envision their health risks, and how do they seek to manage their imagined futures? Moving beyond simplistic pronouncements about race, ethnicity, and culture, these are the crucial questions to consider as we seek to understand the implications of genetic innovation in a diverse society.

What is the appeal of the Dor Yeshorim for Ultra-Orthodox Jews? The key issues continue to be survival, group cohesion, and self-determination. And what can we learn from the controversy in the 1990s over the organization's plans to expand testing from Tay-Sachs to Gaucher's disease and to cystic fibrosis? It reveals that diseases are evolving cultural constructs, symbols with multiple meanings; and it shows how one group's desire for self-determination through disease prevention could be perceived as an attack on the values and prerogatives of those outside the group. The episode also highlights one of the enduring anxieties about the age of genetic medicine: the fear that the more we learn about genetic diseases, the better we get at testing for genetic flaws (in adults, in infants, in fetuses), and the more we embrace "preventive therapy," the more likely it becomes that even the best-intentioned methods of combating genetic disease will mutate into coercive control. Finally, the TSD story highlights the stunning ease with which Americans can racialize identity (using terms like *Jewish genetic disease*), ignoring the profound inadequacies of such concepts and the enormous diversity within groups.[114]

The story of Tay-Sachs disease highlights the many paradoxes of genetic testing for disease prevention. By the 1980s and 1990s, experts acknowledged that prevention was not always the best approach. Writing in the *New England Journal of Medicine* in 1987, one physician acknowledged that prevention was a complex cultural undertaking: "Given some pessimism regarding prevention and the fact that preventive approaches would not be universally acceptable because of differing moral views, what are the prospects for therapy?" He continued, "It is hoped that progress in molecular biology will improve the clinical outlook over the next decade." [115] Such experts looked expectantly toward a future with improved enzyme infusion, transplantation, and gene therapy. Yet the march of prevention would not be halted, stimulating ever more complex controversies. New technologies in embryo manipulation created new dilemmas about the selection of traits in utero. In early 1994, for example, newspapers reported that Virginia physicians working with a Jewish couple had for the first time tested fertilized eggs for Tay-Sachs. Of the four eggs, three "were free of the genetic defect and were implanted in [the woman's] uterus." One developed into a healthy baby. The breakthrough threatened to open another Pandora's box by offering parents a wider selection of traits that verged on enhancement rather than therapy. Asked about this expansion of the prevention approach, ethicist John Fletcher of the University of Virginia voiced concern: "Once you start manipulating genes in the embryo you could move from treating the disease to affecting characteristics that don't have anything to do with the disease, like skin color, height, weight." [116]

As we turn in the next two chapters from Tay-Sachs to cystic fibrosis and sickle cell disease, we see even more clearly how each was traveling its own road, buffeted by different debates over race, ethnicity, and the promise of innovation. These dramatically different therapeutic paths have also reflected distinct notions of risk, group identity, and appropriate therapy, as well as starkly different notions of family and community. The Dor Yeshorim's association of cystic fibrosis with Jewish people in the 1990s high-lighted another tension as well. As Americans were learning of an array of "Jewish genetic diseases," the scientific and popular media widely characterized cystic fibrosis as a "white disease," the most common lethal genetic disease afflicting Caucasians world-wide. The notion that CF was also prevalent among Ashkenazic Jews would have puzzled some Americans. Was CF in fact a "white disease," was it a "Jewish genetic disease," or did it have a broader cultural profile than either term implied? And regardless of who suffered from it and which groups identified with it, was it wise to prevent CF babies from being born when major advances (such as gene therapy) seemed to be just around the corner?

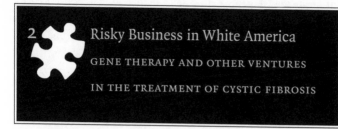

In 1993, people with cystic fibrosis (CF) stood at a crossroads. "Gene Therapy Begins for Fatal Lung Disease," announced the headlines.[1] CF patients could look back over decades of improvements in care that had boosted their life expectancy and forward to the almost unbelievable promise of an imminent cure. Francis Collins, director of the National Human Genome Research Institute and a geneticist who played a key role in identifying the CF gene, was optimistic about the promise of gene therapy. As we saw in chapter 1, he regarded efforts to prevent the birth of CF babies as a "moderate nightmare," especially given the new hope of cure.[2] The architects of the Dor Yeshorim screening program for Tay-Sachs disease had recently suggested expanding the service to include CF, generating a clash of perspectives on the best way to manage such diseases. To be sure, CF was still a deadly genetic disease. Experts who hailed gene therapy in the 1990s often described CF as "the most common fatal inherited disease . . . among Caucasians," using an expansive and vague term to signal the broad reach of the disease across populations of light-skinned peoples.[3] Such seemingly innocuous references to race signaled that this genetic disease belonged to white people more than to others and that cures were on the way.

An elaborate and often contradictory conversation took shape in the 1990s about the links between cystic fibrosis and white, European, or Caucasian identity. Researchers knew that among the staggering number of gene mutations responsible for CF—more than a thousand, by some measures—one particular mutation in the CF gene, called delta F 508 (DF508), accounted for roughly two-thirds of all CF cases.[4] Researchers detected a high prevalence of this gene mutation in geographical Europe, spanning from Algeria to the Netherlands and from Portugal to Turkey, and they theorized that the gene was an index of the prevalence of European, Caucasian, or white genes—making DF508, in their minds, a particularly European gene. Although the mutation accounted for only two-thirds of all CF patients, it became a kind of proxy for studying the transmission of a "European identity." In one South American study, for example, researchers analyzed large variations in DF508 frequency across the region: "The overall frequency . . . in Latin America is 47.7% . . . and 48% in Hispanic patients from USA . . . but it varies from the lowest frequency in Chile (29.2%) up to 62% in Argentina." For them, the variation in DF508 prevalence reflected "different percentages of Caucasian population" across Latin America, with the Argentines presumably being the most European.[5] Such studies slipped effortlessly between seeing DF508 as European, as Caucasian, and as simply a proxy for white.

Was there in fact a clear relationship between cystic fibrosis, the DF508 gene, and white identity? Even across Europe the frequency of the DF508 mutation was remarkably varied. One study suggested that the mutation "shows the highest relative frequency in Denmark (87.2%)."[6] Elsewhere in northern and central Europe the frequency hovered around 72.8 percent. At the same time, however, the percentage in Finland was 46.2 percent, apparently comparable to the rate among Hispanic CF patients in the United States; and in Switzerland the figure was 43.2 percent. If the geographical spread of DF508 was taken seriously as an index of a pure European identity, where would the Swiss and Finnish populations fit within this genetic portrait? The CF gene mutation and CF itself became entangled with different ideas about Europeanness and whiteness in the United States, South America, and elsewhere.[7] Wherever the topic of CF came up, efforts to link the disease through the DF508 mutation to "European" identity resulted in a kind of ethnic myth-making, the creation of diverse narratives about national identity, and in each instance the meanings associated with the term *European* vary widely. Americans, as it turned out, had their own reading of the race issue in CF.

For researchers like Collins, it was not race but the promise of imminent cure that hung heavily in the air in the 1990s. With the detection of genes causing cystic fibrosis, medical researchers looked forward to the day when CF patients—living longer than ever before despite their lung and pancreatic symptoms and their frequent infections—might be cured, relieved once and for all from their condition. A genetics revolution seemed to be under way, and researchers looked askance at the Dor Yeshorim model for preventing CF babies, questioning the idea that preventing such people from ever being born was the optimal solution to genetic disease, especially with the prospect of gene therapy apparently just around the corner.

In the minds of experts like Collins, cystic fibrosis stood at a point quite different from the tragic and always fatal Tay-Sachs disease. By 1993, CF, which had once been a high-mortality childhood disease, seemed increasingly controllable. As people with CF grew through childhood and adolescence and often into adulthood, they coped constantly with heavy mucous secretions that clogged the airways, the gastrointestinal tract, and the ducts of the pancreas, the liver, and the urogenital tract (in males). The mucus caused widespread tissue damage, creating an environment in the lungs where bacteria could multiply too easily. Diabetes was a frequent complication. Digestion was impaired, and patients often succumbed at an early age to lung failure or persistent and overwhelming infections. For many, hospitalization was a common part of life. But over the decades, life expectancy had also risen steadily, so that the child with CF who faced a bleak future in the 1950s would have faced far better odds of making it into adulthood in the 1990s.

Therapeutics was a big part of the reason for this transformation in life chances for people with cystic fibrosis, and in the 1990s, media attention portrayed CF as a disease on the verge of a breakthrough. CF patients seemed to be the most likely to benefit from the advent of a truly novel kind of medicine labeled gene therapy. If the blood-brain barrier stood in the way of delivering on the promise of enzyme replacement for neuropathies like Tay-Sachs disease, with CF it was quite the contrary: the lungs and respiratory system seemed tailor-made for gene therapy, a natural pathway through which a genetically altered virus could deliver new genetic material to ailing parts of the body.[8]

In the mid-1980s, Americans began to hear glowing reports about the prospects of gene therapy, with the great majority supporting the idea.[9] Researchers experimented with different biological agents, documenting the safety and efficacy of specific techniques for transferring genetic material into diseased body parts. It remained to be proven, however, whether this "gene transfer" would remedy the faulty genes responsible for the infirmity. Nevertheless, there was widespread hope that such trials would one day in the near future make gene therapy a reality in hospitals across the nation. National organizations like the Cystic Fibrosis Foundation got behind these efforts. Signs of progress were everywhere. In June 1994 *Discover* magazine noted that cystic fibrosis stood in a special place in the world of gene therapy research. In the search to establish this modality as a viable therapeutic option, "cystic fibrosis may be just the opponent gene therapy has been looking for. It's inherited, it's deadly, and—most important—it's responding."[10] CF was widely seen as a promising "test case" for this experimental practice.[11]

Within a decade, however, the promise of gene therapy faded as gene therapy experiments began to generate their own heated controversies. Viewed in retrospect, the story of cystic fibrosis and gene therapy in the 1990s was a compelling but brief flirtation, an interlude filled with promise as well as with dangers and uncertainties. How should we manage genetic disease? How should we deploy modern genetic knowledge in the name of improving human health? Just as the story of Tay-Sachs disease and the Dor Yeshorim exposed how the management of genetic disease could be deeply entangled with questions of Jewish self-determination and survival, with abortion politics, and with the vagaries of advances in diagnostics, so too did cystic fibrosis become inextricably entangled with its own politics—in this case, the politics of entrepreneurism, business innovation, and hype. To look closely at the history of CF is to explore not only the promise of gene therapy but also the growth of new biotechnology companies and the hopes (and hype) of entrepreneurs who seized on the disease as a way to demonstrate a promising new model of cure for a vast market of patients. The story of CF also makes clear that the advent of gene therapy was part of a longer history of innovation, promise, and risk-taking by patients and their families.

Even as they championed gene therapy, researchers acknowledged that their promises were optimistic and forward-looking. "Twenty years from now," predicted gene therapy pioneer W. French Anderson in 1996, "gene therapy will have revolutionized the practice of medicine. Virtually every disease will have gene therapy as one of its treatments." In particular, cystic fibrosis experts hoped that gene therapy would correct the chloride-transport defect in the lung epithelial cells, a significant problem in the CF patient that results in the buildup of mucus, lung deterioration, infections, and early death. But experts like Anderson admitted that even if successful, gene therapy would be only one among a spectrum of necessary treatments, for CF or any other disease.[12] Despite the public hype, gene therapy would not be a stand-alone cure. Researchers knew that gene therapy could not address some of the typical lung problems in the CF patient and would certainly not repair damaged lung tissue.[13] They knew that using an adenovirus to deliver genetic material to the lungs would not address problems in other parts of the body such as the malabsorption of nutrients, the resulting problems from poor nutrition that were characteristic of CF, and the pancreatic deficiency. They acknowledged that it would not treat the complications — infertility (in males), liver disease, diabetes, or osteoporosis — that sometimes afflict people with CF. Moreover, they also knew that inserting genetically altered viruses into the lungs posed health risks. Yet the promise remained great.

How can the exalted expectations and widely disseminated optimism about gene therapy as a cure for cystic fibrosis be reconciled with the apparent reality that the disease was far too complex for gene therapy alone to tackle effectively? In retrospect it seems that in the best possible scenario, gene therapy would have armed physicians with a new tool to prevent mucus buildup and lung infections in people with CF, possibly extending their lives by decades. It would have been a quantum leap forward in the treatment of the lung problems associated with CF, but not a cure. Nonetheless, during the 1990s gene therapy for CF was frequently portrayed as a cure-all. As one pulmonary specialist noted, "In the next decade, we are going to see a revolution in treatment for this disease. We can really truly think about a cure." [14]

Was the media to blame for this gap between the promise and the likely reality of the gene therapy revolution? The press routinely inflated the curative potential of any new therapy and invariably erred on the side of optimism when reporting on research. Their catering to both professional and lay hopes for a healthier future often came at the expense of accuracy and detail. But we are less concerned with assigning responsibility for the hyperbolic reports than with understanding the historical forces and interests that shaped the hope and the hype. In what follows we look closely at the ideologies and interests that brought patients with cystic fibrosis to this critical and promising juncture. [15]

The willingness of some families, patients, and researchers to embrace the risks associated with this kind of innovation is best understood in a broader historical and cultural context, for their faith in high risks and great rewards stands in sharp contrast to the understandings of risk in the stories of Tay-Sachs disease and (as we shall see) sickle cell disease. Why was this risky therapy elevated in stature at this particular time in professional and popular discourse about CF? Why were ambiguity, confusion, and complexity played down in favor of hype and risk taking? In order to answer such questions, we delve into the long history of cystic fibrosis: the interactions between families and doctors, their emerging shared sense of faith in a steady yet frustrating therapeutic progress, the growing focus on alleviating the deadly lung symptoms of CF, and the ways in which the double-edged advances of antibiotics and transplants laid the groundwork and stoked huge investments in gene therapy.

The gene therapy hype expressed a particular worldview about the transformative possibilities of modern medicine, a worldview that had powerful appeal not just for cystic fibrosis patients and their families but also for pharmaceutical innovators and for the white Americans who were commonly portrayed as the primary victims of the disease. News articles routinely pointed to the disease's impact on majority Americans.[16] Reviewing *Alex*, Frank Deford's 1983 book about his daughter's death from CF, one writer in the *Washington Post* put it this way: "It's a white person's disease, the white version of sickle-cell anemia. It strikes once in every 1,000 live births, and one in twenty whites is a carrier."[17] Deford, an articulate spokesman for the CF cause, represented it as "a genetic disease, carried almost exclusively by Caucasians, but with little fluctuation in incidence anywhere in the white world." This was not quite accurate, for the disease could be found in all parts of the world; but to stress the white or Caucasian character of CF was to obscure its social and demographic complexity. The actual variations mattered little to most readers. Deford concluded, "Apparently it's been with us from antiquity."[18] The message was clear: just as black people had sickle cell disease, white people had cystic fibrosis, a disease that had taken the lead in the race toward gene therapy.

Published in 1983, some six years before scientists had identified and cloned the cystic fibrosis gene, Frank Deford's book about his daughter documented the real-life challenges faced by families and the central role of doctors and drugs in their lives. Massage therapy, regular antibiotics, pneumonia, collapsed lungs, her death at age eight—every detail of the life of Alex Deford as told by her father unfolded in an intimate relationship with the Yale–New Haven hospital system. "Between 1975 and 1976," wrote her father, "when she was going to nursery school and kindergarten . . . [how] innocent I was . . . But at the time the medicines and the treatments kept her on an even keel." [19] At the time, he fully expected that the medicines could continue to keep Alex fit, but in the years afterward his daughter experienced the frequent ups and downs of life with CF.

Through most of its history to date, cystic fibrosis has been understood as a multifaceted problem, not unlike the one portrayed in *Alex*—a problem that called for an intimate and trusting relationship between doctors and parents involved in the care of their children. Yet each generation of patients has experienced CF differently, and families, physicians, and clinical scientists have framed different approaches to it over the years.[20] In contrast with Tay-Sachs disease, the discovery of which dated to the late nineteenth century, CF was a somewhat newer disease. Swiss pediatrician Guido Fanconi and his associates are typically credited with identifying CF in 1936 in their characterization of a group of patients with a "celiac disease" (a digestive disorder). However, it was Dorothy Anderson's 1938 autopsy study of thirty-eight patients at the Babies Hospital in New York City that gave CF its name and, in the words of pioneering researcher Paul di Sant' Agnese, "really put CF on the map as a distinct clinical entity." [21] Anderson described the disease, which she called "cystic fibrosis of the pancreas," as a pancreatic disorder in small children characterized by a severe inability to absorb nutrients and potentially treatable by proper nutrition. This understanding of the disease ushered in the use of dietary supplements and nutritional interventions by families.[22] In the 1940s, antibiotics took center stage, delivering a new tool for managing the infections that afflicted CF patients. In time this would become a critically important improvement, but it would also generate new problems in CF care.

Over time, cystic fibrosis took on many guises. Sidney Farber renamed the disease in the 1940s after uncovering additional features. The new name was *mucoviscidosis*, a term reflecting Farber's understanding of the disease as a systemic one stemming from viscous secretions produced by the mucous glands throughout the body.[23] Nevertheless, diagnosis continued to rely upon identification of pancreatic insufficiency until the mid-1950s. It was then that Paul di Sant' Agnese and his colleagues first noted another feature that became crucial in diagnosis: electrolytes in the sweat of CF patients were elevated.[24] With each discovery came a gradual realization that CF was a complex clinical puzzle and that distinguishing between its primary and secondary features would remain a key conceptual challenge. It was at once a disease of malabsorption, a lung disorder, a pancreatic disease, and a malady defined by an overproduction of mucus.

During the first two decades of its history, cystic fibrosis thus emerged as a multifaceted phenomenon with an ambiguous, but possibly systemic, character. "In light of the 'newness' of the disease," wrote one specialist in 1963, "it is understandable that those who are studying it and caring for patients should not be in full agreement on all aspects."[25] Diagnosis alone was a rapidly evolving practice, with new insights constantly reshaping doctors' ideas about CF's prevalence.

It was only in the 1950s and 1960s that the electrolyte sweat test began to establish that the disease was much more prevalent than previously thought, and only then did the underlying disease afflicting an earlier generation of Alex Defords become visible as such to doctors. A particularly telling article on cystic fibrosis and its treatment appeared in *Time* magazine in 1954. Entitled simply "'New' Disease," the story portrayed CF as a little known child-killer:

> In the wards of Children's Medical Center in Boston last week, or making regular visits to the outpatient clinic, were 2000 youngsters suffering from a mysterious disease with a forbidding name: cystic fibrosis of the pancreas. At Babies Hospital in Manhattan there were seven beds and 80 outpatients; attending Los Angeles' Children's Hospital were 150 known or suspected cases. Across the country are thousands of other victims, most of them probably unrecognized. For to most doctors, pancreatic fibrosis (also known as mucoviscidosis) is a "new" disease.

According to CF specialist Carl Doershuk, this notice in a popular magazine was "undoubtedly the best public relations achievement for CF up to that time."[26] As so often happens, the popularization of the "new" disease along with the new diagnostic test created a rapidly growing population of visible CF patients.

As awareness of this new disease grew, patients, families, and physicians grappled with the multidimensional challenges it posed. What was the emerging picture of the disease? As di Sant' Agnese wrote in 1964, "Most of [the children diagnosed with cystic fibrosis] eventually die in childhood, adolescence, or young adulthood, of the chronic pulmonary involvement which usually dominates the clinical picture and determines the fate of the patient." (From the patient's perspective, the lung problems were the most severe and life threatening aspect of CF.) Physicians were well aware that more and more children with CF were living longer, facing the real possibility of living into their twenties. One study suggested that before 1963, fully half of any cohort of CF sufferers could expect to die within two or three years, but antibiotics, physical therapy drainage, and the use of aerosols had pushed the figure to thirteen or even twenty years. Scientists increasingly understood that a range of new problems would continue to plague these patients as they grew up. As di Sant' Agnese noted, "Despite its name, so-called cystic fibrosis of the pancreas is in reality a generalized disorder" that would pose a continuing and evolving threat to a patient population growing older with the years.[27] In this shifting field much of the professional literature focused on sharpening the diagnostic understanding, developing knowledge of the biochemical bases of CF, and meeting the unfolding challenge of comprehensive management for people with this multidimensional disorder.

By the mid-1960s, cystic fibrosis was no longer "new," nor was it "rare." It had become the subject of increasing public discussion and the focal point of a new comprehensive approach to patient care. As early as 1963 the Cystic Fibrosis Foundation, which had been founded in the early 1950s, promoted "the overriding importance . . . of early diagnosis and prompt institution of a complex and comprehensive care regimen."[28] According to the Matthews Comprehensive Treatment Program—first developed in the 1950s and increasingly the standard in the 1960s—ideal CF care would involve an array of specialists and would place the patient and family at the center of a program of aggressive disease management, with a strong focus on anticipating and preventing problems.[29] This ideal of comprehensive care was driven not only by the national organization, but by the changing relationship between patients, families, and caregivers. Perhaps most crucial, it required that the family become intimately involved in day-to-day care.

Comprehensive care also required resources, and to some extent it was made possible by the broadening social commitments of these years. As historians have noted, the 1960s were a time when patients, families, regulators, and politicians were all pressing for attention to the wide-ranging challenges posed by a host of new health problems from cancer to kidney failure. Increasingly, patients demanded responsiveness to the social and psychological dimensions of illness as well as to the biological aspects.[30]

In CF, the Cystic Fibrosis Foundation became a key force advocating for patients and families. These pressures to focus on the patient's and family's perspective continued to grow in the 1970s and 1980s, at times in subtle conflict with the aims of CF researchers and practitioners. Nevertheless, the creation, as early as 1960, of medical centers specifically devoted to cystic fibrosis points to the power of this disease to command resources that were unavailable to other groups.[31]

According to the comprehensive care model, parents were the primary caregivers in the front lines of disease management. For example, the 1963 Cystic Fibrosis Foundation's *Guide to Diagnosis and Management* characterized therapeutics as supplementary to home care. This and other such handbooks suggested that therapeutic interventions carried out in the home—whether specialized mist tent therapies, postural drainage of mucus, coaching children in breathing exercises, or encouraging them in their physical activity—were of crucial importance; and these practices helped shape parents' appreciation for what therapeutic innovations could mean for their children.[32] Other studies suggested that lifestyle, exercise, sleep patterns, breathing and lung capacity as well as family relationships could all shape the patient's experience. Such concerns about the cystic fibrosis experience would dominate medical and scientific writing from the 1960s onward.

Facing the formidable challenges of in-home care for babies and young children with cystic fibrosis, parents turned to physicians for coaching and came to see therapeutic innovation as their friend and partner. Clinical centers offered a specialized resource-rich brand of what parents were encouraged to do at home. As one article noted, "When a physician embarks on the treatment of a child with cystic fibrosis, he simultaneously undertakes the treatment and involvement of the entire family." Family medicine was just beginning to take shape as a subspecialty, and the direction of CF care meshed neatly with this trend. As the article continued, "This current view maintains that the family of the CF child has to be enlisted actively in the overall treatment and therapeutic planning for the child and integrated into a smoothly functioning team."[33] Patients, physicians, and parents were part of the same team, sharing a common perspective—this idea was central to CF care in the 1970s. And this standard of care was being realized, for more and more patients, precisely because of the resources available in the comprehensive care setting. Handbooks and studies emphasized that this style of care was crucial because of the complex nature of CF. The best therapy, it was said, involved securing the cooperation of child and parent, "since both child and parent carry an unusual responsibility for the patient's well-being."[34]

Throughout the following decades comprehensive care would be hailed as the single most important factor in the dramatic improvement in the life expectancy and health of people with cystic fibrosis.[35] Meanwhile, research studies produced better methods of dealing with the daily task of clearing airways of mucus.[36] Other studies examined the pros and cons of different agents for breaking up lung sputum.[37] Yet others explored the changing lifestyle challenges faced by CF patients as they became older, touching upon problems of reproduction and fertility.[38] By the 1970s, such advances alongside intensive home-based care had made it possible for more and more CF children to live into adolescence and adulthood.[39] Indeed, chapter after chapter of Frank Deford's *Alex* testifies to the intense involvement of families in day-to-day care. Deford recalled, for example, that even though he was skeptical about the benefits, he administered postural drainage therapy perhaps two thousand times in eight years, his wife even more.[40] In every disease, a particular doctor-patient-family relationship takes shape. In each case, a particular ethos evolves. In the history of cystic fibrosis, comprehensive management was a major cultural development, a key factor shaping sentiments and future expectations about medical innovation and establishing a framework for how doctors, patients, and families thought about their relationship with each other.

Who were these cystic fibrosis patients and families? Did they have an ethnic or racial profile? And what were the key aspects of their experiences? The road from comprehensive care to CF gene therapy involved many shifts in scientific thinking and much political debate about who these patients were and which aspects of the disease were the most important. Whereas medical scientists in the 1960s understood CF first and foremost as a comprehensive and systemic problem, in the age of gene therapy the disease came to be considered primarily in terms of its genetic and pulmonary features. These two different understandings highlight the cultural perceptions of two different eras not only about why CF patients were dying but about who they were—white, black, or multiethnic.

In the 1960s and 1970s, even as comprehensive management focused researchers, clinicians, patients, and their families on an imposing array of clinical challenges, scientists often disagreed about the primary character of cystic fibrosis.[41] Raising a child with CF from infancy through adolescence continued to be a formidable undertaking. Neither families nor experts emphasized the "genetic" features of the disease. To be sure, they understood it to be a "hereditary" disorder, but this way of thinking did not capture what they saw as its fundamental biological underpinnings. Rather, scientists strongly believed that the disease needed to be addressed at the metabolic and biochemical level—that is, that mucus buildup throughout the body was the crucial and primary issue, and that underlying biochemical abnormalities were responsible for the systemic problem. The age of comprehensive care dictated that there would be considerable doubt about the wisdom of giving precedence to one feature of CF over others, or for that matter of thinking of the disorder principally as a "lung disease."

According to the prevailing view, studying the underlying mechanisms of mucus accumulation would "contribute to a more fundamental understanding of the clinical problem."[42] Therefore, throughout the 1950s and 1960s, researchers at the National Institutes of Health (NIH) tried to unravel the mysteries of cystic fibrosis by studying "the basic biochemical, biophysical and physiological disturbances implicated." The research agenda addressed three features: the "triad of chronic pulmonary disease, pancreatic deficiency and abnormally high sweat electrolytes." As Paul di Sant' Agnese put it, "In patients with cystic fibrosis there is a ready-made experimental model in which to study the interaction between mucopolysaccharides and electrolytes." In this view, CF research was driven by the assumption that these biochemical substances and their interaction were the underlying keys to the puzzle of the disease. The research findings would reach far beyond the "fight against CF," di Sant' Agnese observed, since studies on the disease "may also help to answer some of the unsolved questions of physiology, with broad implications in human pathology."[43] For such researchers, then, CF was part of a broader research agenda; and there was a powerful sense that studying the underlying mechanisms of biochemical imbalances in the body, abnormal mucus production, and organ damage in CF would be applicable to CF patient care as well as to general questions in physiology and metabolic disease.

But research agendas and ideas about the true nature of the disorder were also shaped by politics and by the competition for resources. Many diseases vied for public attention and federal resources in the early 1970s. Legislative debate swirled over a wide range of medical issues, from national health insurance to the war on cancer. Sickle cell disease legislation (to address a hereditary disease associated with African Americans) was winding its way through Congress en route to President Nixon's desk for signing. Such "ethnic" diseases as Tay-Sachs and sickle cell disease had taken on powerful cultural and political meanings. Debates about funding often turned into arguments about national research priorities and about privilege, equality, and fairness in addressing the concerns of diverse groups in America.

Increasing legislative interest in disease and health in the 1970s introduced a political angle to the question of what cystic fibrosis was, whom it affected, and how research should be carried out. Indeed, when Congress took up legislation in 1972 to increase research funding for heart, lung, blood vessel, and blood disorders, CF became part of this larger political discussion. One question that emerged was whether cystic fibrosis was a "lung disorder" entitled to funding under this bill. Or was it best understood as a "metabolic disorder"? Was it a *white* disease or a *panethnic* concern? In this context, some critics suggested, the scientific community's focus on electrolytes, mucopolysaccharides, and underlying mechanisms seemed far removed from the practical concerns of families and patients.

Legislators heard testimony from a number of researchers, and the politicized atmosphere revealed that the multidimensional disease could mean very different things to different people. Some researchers insisted that cystic fibrosis should not be included in lung disease legislation because, as one physician put it, "the disease is a metabolic disorder and the biochemical disturbance which is responsible for the clinical manifestations [is] not confined to the lungs."[44] This view, which was the standard research view, was seconded by NIH director Robert Marston, who insisted that extensive research on CF was already being supported by the National Institute of Arthritis and Metabolic Diseases.[45] Only four years earlier, in 1968, legislation had provided strong support for comprehensive pulmonary care facilities around the country, which everyone acknowledged had benefited cystic fibrosis patients greatly.

Indeed, some observers regarded cystic fibrosis as a relatively privileged disease. For example, during the legislative hearings regarding research funds for sickle cell disease, advocates for the new program had pointed to the vast discrepancies between private funding for CF and for sickle cell disease. As one researcher noted, "In 1967, there were an estimated 1,155 new cases of [sickle cell] disease, 1,206 of cystic fibrosis, 813 of muscular dystrophy . . . Yet volunteer organizations raised $1.9 million for cystic fibrosis and $7.9 million for muscular dystrophy, but less than $100,000 for sickle cell anemia."[46] So as Congress debated the new Heart, Lung, Blood Vessel, and Blood Bill in 1972, advocates for CF found themselves competing for attention with various disadvantaged-disease constituencies. Clearly, if cystic fibrosis was to hold on to existing support and secure further funding under the new legislation, advocates would have to readjust its image as a privileged disease and also recharacterize its fundamental biology.

Dr. Giulio Barbero, a CF physician at the University of Pennsylvania and a spokesman for the National Cystic Fibrosis Research Foundation, understood the need for such a reframing at a time like this, when the major government initiative that had provided funding for pulmonary disease programs, including CF care, faced cutbacks. In his testimony before the House subcommittee, Barbero disputed the prevailing characterization of the disease as articulated by NIH director Robert Marston. He insisted that cystic fibrosis was one among a spectrum of "children's lung diseases . . . [in which] many contributing causes, genetic and non-genetic, known and unknown, are involved." It would be, he argued, "unsound to separate out cystic fibrosis . . . It is a lung disease," and as such it warranted funding under the new legislation.[47] This depiction of CF was at once opportunistic and pragmatic. It focused on what patients and families believed to be the most important aspect of the disease, as opposed to the underlying mechanisms that preoccupied scientists.

In making his appeal, however, Barbero reduced the symptomatological complexity of cystic fibrosis to a caricature. His argument transformed one of the central clinical manifestations of the disease—its devastating pulmonary problems—into the only problem: "Cystic fibrosis is the most serious pulmonary disease of man; it acts as a key model in understanding the research aspects for pulmonary disease, and therefore must exist in some juxtaposition to the spectrum of understanding . . . pulmonary disease in man."[48] Speaking for the Cystic Fibrosis Foundation, whose lobbying efforts had always been strong, and to some extent for patients, Barbero implied that the tendency of researchers to characterize CF as "a metabolic disorder and a biochemical disturbance" was far too rigid, too removed from clinical realities and the actual experience of the disease.[49] In the end, his argument persuaded legislators to focus on the patient's experiences rather than on the scientific questions stressed in testimony from the NIH establishment figures, and CF was covered under the new funding. Not surprisingly, at that very moment the Cystic Fibrosis Foundation was promoting its 1972 poster child as a "lung-damaged" patient living with the burden of a fatal inherited disorder.[50]

Barbero's testimony touched on all the themes that would continue to be part of the reframing of cystic fibrosis—its biology, its true demographics, its impact on families and children, the proper research agenda for the disease, and the growing role of funding agencies and financial interests in establishing this agenda—with one telling difference: he chose to emphasize the *panethnic* rather than the *white* face of cystic fibrosis. In his testimony Barbero compared CF with another newly politicized high-profile disease, sickle cell disease (SCD). Only months earlier SCD had gained national attention as a hereditary disorder prevalent in African-American communities. Congress was preparing to pass the National Sickle Cell Anemia Control Act to provide funding for treatment, research, and counseling for SCD patients and families.[51] In this context, Barbero reminded lawmakers that CF carriers were more prevalent than SCD carriers, and he emphasized that CF was also a significant concern in the black population. He did not present it as a "Caucasian" disease, as scientists would do in the 1980s and 1990s. Such a framing would not have resonated in the political atmosphere of the early 1970s as it did in later years. Thus, Barbero highlighted that while 5 percent of the total population were CF carriers, 2 percent of the black population were CF carriers.[52]

In the 1970s, when many Americans were focusing on remedies for racial injustice and the disenfranchisement of African Americans, physicians and advocates for cystic fibrosis patients chose not to publicly frame it as a "white" disease. The choice is hardly surprising. Such terminology would have done little to mobilize public support and legislative sympathy in a decade when the political impetus was to remedy the effects of racial and social privilege. The push was on for national health insurance, for legislation to make kidney dialysis more accessible to all Americans, to fund research and health care for sickle cell disease and for thalassemia (prevalent among Greek and Italian Americans), and so on. In this context, though many acknowledged the high rates of CF among white Americans, advocates also highlighted its more complex ethnic profile.[53] A long list of articles explored manifestations of the disease in black Americans and in other ethnic and nonwhite groups.[54] The cultural framing of CF, in the 1970s as in the 1990s, was sensitive to the social and cultural context of the times.

Over the following decades, political, scientific, and clinical agendas as well as patients' concerns would continue to reframe cystic fibrosis. Though the argument that CF was a lung disease was clearly part of a political effort to bring CF under the umbrella of the 1972 legislation, in subsequent years the lung problems associated with the disease would become increasingly central in research and therapeutic management, particularly as the patient population matured and grew in numbers.

Where would cystic fibrosis research and patient care go from here? CF therapy was situated at a complex intersection in the 1970s. On one side were the new concerns of a maturing patient group; on another side were different research paradigms that tried to reduce the disease's complexity to simple models; and on yet another side were emerging business concerns bent on marketing innovative cures that pushed the limits of CF care. It is with these forces in mind that we can understand the impact and meaning of three other innovations—antibiotic regimens, lung transplantations, and gene therapy—that would shape popular thinking about CF in the years between 1970 and 2000. Each modality had its particular impact on patients' lives and expectations. Each one also reflected the agendas of CF specialists who were constantly refining their understanding of the biology of the disease and their ideas about how best to help the patients and families. As the stories of antibiotics, lung transplants, and gene therapy unfolded, however, they also revealed the ambiguities of therapeutic innovation and the sometimes dramatic collision between patient expectations, scientific research agendas, and business interests.

TRADING ONE DISEASE FOR ANOTHER: ANTIBIOTICS, TRANSPLANTATION, AND FRUSTRATING PROGRESS ON THE ROAD TO GENE THERAPY

For much of the history of cystic fibrosis, progress also brought frustrations. Constant improvements in CF care, from antibiotic therapy to lung transplantation, bettered the situation of patients. Yet the advances always seemed to be mixed blessings, ushering in new challenges such as antibiotic-resistant organisms or extensive after-transplant health problems. Over time, these advances also threatened to ensnare patients and researchers in economic and ethical entanglements. Increasing longevity too brought new challenges. The frustrations of progress became a key part of the sensibility of CF patients and doctors, shaping how they weighed therapeutic risks and how they embraced innovations like gene therapy. Progress had been imperfect, they reasoned, but a cure was ultimately achievable. It was a conceit that contrasted sharply with current notions surrounding the cure of people with Tay-Sachs disease and, as we shall see, people with sickle cell disease.

Beginning with the widespread production of penicillin and the advent of synthetic antibacterial agents in the mid-1940s and 1950s, antibiotics assumed a central and problematic role in the treatment of cystic fibrosis. Perceived as a revolutionary medicine, antibiotics allowed physicians to tackle a wide range of the bacterial infections that manifested themselves as pulmonary congestion in CF patients, including pneumonia and tuberculosis. But as early as 1951 three researchers noted that "the enlarged chemical and antibiotic armamentarium of the physician today has brought increasing clinical importance to the *Pseudomonas* strain of organisms at all ages." The drugs provided relief from lung infections but also promoted the growth of resistant organisms. The authors continued, invoking simple laws of biology: "Any regimen of long-continued therapy with a single antibacterial agent invites the development of highly resistant organisms which may flourish in an environment rendered more favorable by the absence of susceptible bacteria."[55] Thus, even as penicillin and other drugs assumed an expanding role in CF management, physicians were becoming aware of the risks posed by these powerful new weapons.

From the outset, antibacterial therapy was a balancing act for the clinician. Therapy was a subtle negotiation: use enough of the drug to combat the infectious organisms that often colonize the thick mucus in the lungs of CF patients, but not enough to encourage the proliferation of the more resistant bacterial strains. In 1968, with an ever-increasing array of antibiotics coming onto the market, researchers pointed out that the heavy use of penicillin had produced a new bacterial problem: "There is little doubt that the establishment of [*Pseudomonas aeruginosa*] in the respiratory tract is encouraged by suppression of other bacteria by antibiotics."[56] The struggle to control this bacterial strain was fast becoming a fact of life for more and more CF patients. As Frank Deford put it, "For all the research that has been done, there is as yet no antibiotic to deal with pseudomonas, and once it begins to march through the lungs, it multiplies with impunity and sweeps everything in its path."[57] Nevertheless, the trend toward the use of more antibiotics, in increasing varieties, continued into the late 1970s.[58]

The problem was not the drugs, of course, but the way doctors and patients had been using them. In the 1960s and early 1970s, assessments of antibacterial therapies were few in number, and they were largely anecdotal and retrospective.[59] The use of antibiotics to treat CF had "been more of a ritual . . . than a scientific approach."[60] In the late 1970s, however, researchers began to scrutinize these therapies more rigorously, and a new therapeutic approach evolved. Instead of using a single preferred antibiotic, practitioners began to alternate among different agents, timing their interventions carefully so as to keep bacteria "off balance" and weighing the various agents (wide spectrum, narrow spectrum, oral, intravenous, etc.) against one another.

A tension regarding antibacterial care for cystic fibrosis arose just as a new face of the CF patient was emerging. The disease now affected growing numbers of adolescents and adults who had survived their early years as CF children. It was also rising in prevalence, partly because new screening techniques were identifying more patients. And it was attaining a higher social and political profile, thanks to the 1972 Heart, Lung, Blood Vessel, and Blood Bill as well as the 1976 Genetic Disease Act. The number of patients receiving care had more than doubled in ten years (from an estimated 4,523 in 1965 to 10,489 in 1976).[61] Doctors in this period documented significant variation within this clinical population, as well as significant differences in patients' responses to antibacterial therapies, physiotherapy, and other therapeutics. Amid this veritable explosion of treatment options, how was one to determine the actual efficacy of antibacterial therapies? As one author noted in 1978, "While it is accepted by many that the increased longevity of CF patients is strongly related to antibiotic use, this has never been documented adequately."[62]

Were antibiotics the magic sword of CF care? Or was the sword double-edged in some way? In the 1970s and early 1980s, numerous clinical trials were undertaken to determine the actual effect of various antibiotics on pulmonary exacerbations (severe and acute attacks) in CF patients. For example, the introduction of ticarcillin (a semisynthetic penicillin derivative) prompted a comparative study of three particular alternatives: "ticarcillin alone, ticarcillin plus gentamicin, and gentamicin alone in [twenty-eight] patients with CF."[63] The scientific presumption of this period was that the only way to control extreme variations in clinical care was the double-blind placebo-controlled crossover study.[64] The imperative to do highly structured clinical trials seemed obvious to researchers looking back over decades of drug innovation and trying to evaluate wide variations in CF management. They questioned the impressionistic basis on which doctors reported their failures and successes in antibacterial therapy for CF.[65] They saw themselves to some extent as reformers standing in judgment on acute care and routine clinical practice, looking at dosing implications and interactions among antibiotics.[66] Antibiotics had created a brave new world of medical care, but one that needed to be rationalized. The clinical trials of the late 1970s and early 1980s set out to bring order to the increasing biological and clinical complexity of CF and to help practitioners sort through the drugs available for treating acute pulmonary exacerbations in CF patients.

Many within this generation of researchers remained cautious about the promise of breakthroughs or cures. Understanding that even "miracle drugs" like antibiotics had their perils, they felt that one goal of clinical research should be to regulate the use of innovative drugs—a position sharply opposed to that of the research entrepreneurs who would later take up the torch of gene therapy. The new clinical trials on antibiotic therapies served a slightly different function from earlier research on the disease's underlying mechanisms or research on the family's role in CF care. Although this antibiotics research was aimed at a rather limited problem in clinical practice, it impinged nevertheless on a complex set of social problems: how to cope with pharmacological abundance, how to discipline individualism in medical practice, how to prevent the overuse of antibiotics, and how best to serve the increasingly adolescent cohort of CF patients who were altering the balance of family-centered care.

In the mid-1980s, as they looked back on the evolution of antibacterial therapy for cystic fibrosis, physicians and researchers recognized that antibiotics were a double-edged sword. Some researchers, in view of the side effects of such "drugs of choice," called for research into newer antibacterial drugs.[67] Others expressed concern about the hypersensitivity of some CF patients to semisynthetic penicillin.[68] Still others pointed to the role of antibiotics in the evolution of disturbing new infections in CF patients, such as the increasing frequency of a new *Pseudomonas* infection (*P. cepacia*) that posed even more formidable challenges than *P. aeruginosa*.[69] Some even questioned the basic premises and efficacy of antibacterial therapy, proposing that antibiotic therapy was not as important as intensive chest physiotherapy in CF management.[70]

In 1985, the pediatrician John Nelson commented perceptively on the ironies of progress in CF care and the frustrating problems that had been created by the sheer abundance of new drugs. If privilege and abundance had any downsides, this was one of them. "Historically," he explained, "patients with cystic fibrosis have been given a variety of prophylactic regimens. It was very common at one time to give tetracycline for a few months, then chloramphenicol for a few months, and then other drugs for a few months." This regimen created an impression of control and progress, and "patients were reported to do better [even though] controlled studies were not done." Although clinical trials tried to remedy inconsistencies in care, many physicians continued to resist standardization—and for good reasons. The complexity of the disease and its variability from one patient to the next guaranteed that no single mode of therapy would ever be established as a standard in CF antibacterial care. The "objective" guidance offered by clinical drug trials could not dispel the difficulties of managing the increasing biological complexity of CF. "The issue is still clouded," said Nelson. He, like many other physicians, understood well the limits of antibiotics and clinical trials and looked forward to new approaches. He mused, "Perhaps when the basic defect in cystic fibrosis is understood, the relationship of the host to the microorganism will be better understood." Implicit in such remarks was a quiet yearning for a breakthrough, perhaps even a genetic breakthrough, as CF care moved away from staged prophylactic regimens.[71]

Increasingly, researchers conceived of cystic fibrosis as a respiratory disease, and their focus on antibiotics reinforced that trend. The antibiotics revolution also introduced doctors to the numerous drug companies with high economic stakes in CF care. Certainly there were some researchers who held on to traditional views of CF, arguing that "the pulmonary disease in CF was secondary to the pancreatic deficiency."[72] But by the 1980s that concept had been pushed into the background. Concerns about antibacterial agents had also brought researchers into close relationships with representatives of the pharmaceutical industry, the makers and marketers of these new products. Years later, when the focus shifted to gene therapy, this relationship would advance a step further: researchers would frequently become part of the drug development team, acting as interested and invested intermediaries between patients and families, on one hand, and drug production companies on the other. But for now, as frustrations with the therapeutic status quo grew in the 1980s, another group of specialists—the transplant surgeons—were busily promoting their own revolution in CF care. The embrace of lung transplantation represented yet another feature of the gradual reinvention of CF as a pulmonary disease.

The champions of lung transplantation looked back on the era of antibiotics and concluded that the therapeutic gains for cystic fibrosis had run their course: progress had leveled off. "Aggressive palliative therapy remains the basis of treatment," noted one article in 1991. "However . . . the plateau has probably been reached, and we need innovative treatments."[73] Transplantation seemed to point the way to the future of CF care, particularly in view of the extended life span and new dilemmas facing people with CF. "The median survival age in 1989 was 26 years, compared to only 7 years in 1964," noted one researcher. "The extended survival is due in part to more aggressive treatment of pulmonary disease and malnutrition." Having succeeded in bringing increased numbers of CF children into young adulthood, physicians and patients confronted the new reality that "pulmonary disease remains the primary cause of morbidity and mortality in noninfant CF patients."[74] Fatal lung infections had come to be the most fearful reality of the disease.

To call cystic fibrosis a pulmonary disease was to focus, ever more persistently, on remedies for lung deterioration. Despite the gastrointestinal, pancreatic, and liver problems associated with the disease, the lungs drew disproportionate attention from the 1970s onward. The reason was clear: increasingly, it was lung problems that ultimately killed CF patients. Advances in antibacterial medicine had increased families' expectations but had not diminished their desperation. In this context, radical therapeutic gambits like lung transplantation could emerge as a viable option for CF patients in the mid-1980s, promising new lives and healthy lungs for ailing patients. "Lung transplantation" in fact comprised a diverse array of innovative surgical procedures, among them single-lung, double-lung, and heart-lung transplantation. The story of lung transplantation in cystic fibrosis provides further insight into how the threat of death still loomed over CF patients and their families, and how patients often embraced more daring therapeutic opportunities despite the risks.

From the start, transplantation was a bold and risky proposition. Transplant medicine boomed in the 1980s in the wake of the discovery of immunosuppressive drugs to prevent rejection of new organs.[75] The first heart-lung transplantation (HLT) in 1981 set the stage for future lung transplantations in CF. At the time, as one author noted, concerns were voiced about the applicability of HLT to cystic fibrosis: "Enthusiasm . . . was initially tempered by consideration of a number of potential problems unique to the CF patient." Among these were concerns that the CF defect might recur in the newly transplanted lungs. There was also concern that immunosuppression would result in postoperative respiratory infections, and that control of the diabetes that was common to CF patients would be made more difficult by post-transplantation steroid therapy. Of course, match donor organs—truly a scarce commodity—also had to be found. Despite the difficulties, in 1984 a surgical team at the University of Pittsburgh undertook the first heart-lung transplantation in a CF patient. The effort failed, but it encouraged surgeons at other centers to try similar lung transplant interventions.[76]

The HLT enterprise expanded rapidly from the mid-1980s through the 1990s, bringing significant new income to health centers around the nation. The advent of cyclosporine A, an immunosuppressive drug that helped prevent rejection of the implanted organs, had ushered in this new era for transplantation. The high price of transplants made the enterprise a lucrative one. At first, the cost of heart-lung transplants ranged from $75,000 to $125,000, and insurers balked at paying such staggering expenses.[77] But as insured Americans pushed companies to pay, academic health centers came to see transplant medicine as a crucial tool in building revenue, retaining preeminence in research and health care, and becoming competitive in economically difficult times.[78]

Transplantation reinforced the idea that the lung was the central therapeutic challenge in cystic fibrosis, but the transplant option also focused attention on the painful end-of-life crises confronting patients with severe lung deterioration. Decade by decade, the maturing of the CF patient had pushed these issues out of pediatrics and into the realm of adolescent and adult medicine, where decisions about end-of-life care, risky therapeutics, and the pros and cons of treatment options were approached very differently. Only a decade or so earlier, therapeutics had been shaped by the challenges of rearing a child with cystic fibrosis.[79] But by the early 1990s, CF patients were now more often independent adults grappling with profound concerns and willing to take significant risks. Parents too seemed increasingly willing to incur greater risks for their children with CF.

In 1991 Stanley Fiel noted of transplantation, "There is now a therapeutic option for end-stage CF that points up how the field has moved beyond the stark antinomy of heroics versus palliation." In other words, in the past when physicians and patients faced the end-of-life realities of CF, they typically thought either in fatalistic terms (hospice) or in heroic terms (last-ditch interventions). But transplantation, he insisted, was a third kind of option, neither fatalistic nor heroic: damaged lungs were simply replaced with healthy donor organs in an effort to extend the lives of CF patients. In 1991, in view of the growing number of transplant cases and the apparent fact "that the transplanted lungs do not redevelop CF," Fiel called the use of HLT in cystic fibrosis "an example of what now may provisionally be called a therapeutic breakthrough in a chronic disease." Of course, no one claimed that HLT would alter the "pervasiveness and progressive course of the disease." Fiel and many other authors, though optimistic, typically framed their evaluations as "provisional," based on "apparent" and "potential" facts—and rightly so, since the cases were few in number and the long-term implications remained unclear.[80] Though transplant surgeons might hope that the biology of the disease could be significantly altered by lung transplantation, they acknowledged that mortality depended upon a variety of extrapulmonary factors, among them nutrition, pancreatic disorder, and infection.

Professional and popular writers invested enormous hope in this daring technique even as they acknowledged its limitations. An article in *Time* magazine noted, "Experts on cystic fibrosis agree . . . that such surgical wonders are of limited use . . . for transplantation was not appropriate for all CF patients, since many suffer from diabetes, kidney failure and other complications that make them ineligible for transplants." In fact, in the best circumstances transplantation could serve only a small percentage of CF patients, since "a shortage of lung donors poses an even greater problem."[81] Some public media focused on the "life-giving" possibilities of lung transplantation.[82] But most popular articles in the late 1980s and early 1990s conceded that lung transplants in cystic fibrosis were a "last resort," a dramatic, risky gambit at the end stage of the disease. *People* magazine reported, "Complications of the transplant itself—rejection of the lungs, or infection—can be fatal."[83]

If lung transplantation represented a major crossroads in CF care in the 1980s and 1990s, it was still a complex problem that revealed the administrative, sociological, and economic difficulties of bringing high-tech medicine within reach of all Americans. It was an option primarily for those with insurance coverage, or those with the money to pay out of pocket. It was also a socially complex enterprise relying on donor networks to make scarce organs available. Transplantation meant long wait times and highlighted the connectedness of patients via the vast organ-sharing network. And it involved continuous medical care after the operation in order to combat organ rejection, care that entailed significant health risks of its own. In short, transplantation, like comprehensive care, required resources—even more resources, in fact. Transplantation also involved complex processes with major impediments to success, and it meant lifelong post-transplant medical care.

Experts insisted that heart-lung transplantation, a particularly complex, expensive procedure, should not be considered a cure, regardless of the popular hype. Rather, it was a tradeoff with its own set of dangers and frustrations. "I don't think you can call organ transplantation a cure," noted surgeon Thomas Spray in 1992, after almost a decade of performing transplant operations on CF patients. "It will extend the life of patients," he affirmed, but the need for regular medical care throughout post-transplant life meant that patients were simply "trading one kind of disease for another. Having a transplant is a chronic illness."[84]

There was something else noteworthy about lung transplantation: it was, for the most part, an unregulated and entrepreneurial kind of innovation, and it involved some of the most extensive high-tech teamwork in medicine. As lung transplantation for cystic fibrosis expanded at academic health centers during the 1980s and 1990s, it became part of the unfolding story of for-profit health care. These surgical centers were largely unfettered by government regulation or sweeping institutional oversight, because surgical innovation had never fallen under the purview of the Food and Drug Administration (FDA). Innovation in transplant surgery was not controlled by the same regulatory procedures that evaluated and controlled the market in drugs, and as such it was surrounded by an air of entrepreneurism.[85] Patients, families, and practitioners worked together to locate donors, to negotiate with insurers about payment, and to find surgeons capable of carrying out the expensive procedures. One author, voicing a concern raised by many others, wondered, "Should resources be devoted to rather exotic procedures [like HLT] benefiting a few rather than to more ordinary measures that may help many people?"[86] This was an emerging dilemma throughout the American health care system in the 1980s and 1990s, a time of intense debate about the nation's health priorities, about privilege and injustice, about the virtues of deregulation, and about the embrace of costly high-technology medicine over basic care.

Thus, in the 1990s, at the dawn of the age of gene therapy for cystic fibrosis, experts spoke of both promise and frustration, and many of them looked anxiously for new breakthroughs that might finally carry CF patients into the promised land of cure. As CF researchers and patients looked back on the history of comprehensive care, antibiotics, and lung transplantation, they saw therapeutic progress, they saw sick children living longer and becoming young adults, and they also saw unexpected side effects and health setbacks. Patients had in many respects traded one type of deadly disease for another—one that was manageable, but still deadly. The appeal of gene therapy in CF must be seen in the light of these earlier therapeutic and social developments. Physicians and researchers looked at the aging population of CF patients and saw frustration with both antibacterial therapy and lung transplantation, and a willingness to take bold risks in the face of death. Patients and their families looked at researchers and saw an entrepreneurial ethos that championed risk taking and hope; an increasing focus on the lungs as the critical organ in CF care; and a research culture that embraced innovation and increasingly turned practitioners, surgeons, and scientists into salesmen and entrepreneurs. And all these groups saw a poignant disease that some white Americans had come to identify as their own.

A DARING VENTURE FOR THE RISKTAKERS: GENE THERAPY IN THE 1990S

In the 1990s, at the very time when questions about lung transplantation and antibiotic medicine for cystic fibrosis were roiling the profession, gene therapy emerged as a wonderous dream, a scientific fantasy inspiring intense hope, despite the risks. "We're hoping," said Robert Beall of the Cystic Fibrosis Foundation, "that two new drug therapies, plus gene therapy in the near future, will someday prevent the need for lung transplants."[87] Gene therapy quickly attracted both public and professional acclaim as a revolutionary innovation for CF and other diseases. The reaction was extraordinarily optimistic, especially for an experimental procedure that had produced no proven benefits to any patient with any disease. There was, however, good reason for optimism. The excitement about gene therapy followed on the heels of the discovery in 1989 of one of the defective genes implicated in CF, a discovery made possible by extensive investment in mapping the human genome and identifying disease-causing genes.[88] This defective gene apparently resulted in the failure of chloride to pass through the walls of cells in the CF patient, a failure that led to mucus accumulation, lung deterioration, and early death. Gene therapy was hypothetically envisioned as a method of repairing the chloride transport process by somehow inserting corrective copies of the newly discovered gene into the tissue in the lungs. In championing gene therapy for lung repair, its advocates adopted the prevailing lung-oriented assumptions about the disease. But

Cystic Fibrosis

"THE MOST COMMON FATAL INHERITED
DISEASE AMONG CAUCASIANS"

Understanding of CF has evolved rapidly in the last four decades, thanks to novel scientific ideas, therapeutic innovations, and CF's increasing cultural significance in America.

Carrier Frequency	1 in 25–30 Caucasians and Ashkenazic Jews
Disease Incidence	1 in 2,500–4,500 Caucasians
Life Expectancy	Mid-thirties (median); over 40 percent of U.S. patients are adults
Inheritance	Autosomal recessive
Cause	Gene mutation on chromosome 7; over 1,000 CF mutations identified
Mechanism	By current accounts, CF begins as a defective gene known as the CF transmembrane conductance regulator (CFTR), which allows the body to produce thick, sticky mucous secretions that affect various organ systems. Most seriously, the mucus clogs the lungs, leading to life-threatening lung infections, or it obstructs the pancreas and prevents proper food absorption and digestion.
Symptoms	The symptoms of CF vary widely from one patient to another, and include salty-tasting skin; thick sputum; persistent coughing; wheezing or shortness of breath; chronic lung infections; weight loss; greasy, bulky stools; nasal polyps; and sterility among males. Long-term complications include lung failure, stress on cardiovascular system, and diabetes.
Diagnosis	There are many methods for diagnosing CF, from a simple sweat test to more

	complicated tests that can identify specific gene mutations. A high concentration of salt in the patient's sweat indicates CF.
Treatments	CF is manageable, but treatments are as diverse as the disease itself and have been central to transforming the CF experience over the last several decades. These include clearing mucus from the lungs, chest physical therapy (including vigorous back clapping), aerosolized antibiotics used to treat lung infections, mucus-thinning drugs, antibiotics for chronic infections, and pancreatic enzymes and strict diets for digestive and nutritional issues. Lung transplantation is available for patients with lung failure.
Prevention	Prenatal testing for fetuses is possible using amniocentesis or chorionic villi sampling to identify the CF gene. Carrier testing is available for adults.

Since its discovery in the late-1930s, CF has been transformed from a fatal childhood disease into a chronic but manageable disease. Screening programs have curbed the incidence of the disease.[*] It is estimated, however, that over ten million Americans carry the CF gene.

[*]Jeanette E. Dankert-Roelse and Gerard J. Te Meerman, "Screening for Cystic Fibrosis: Time to Change Our Position?" *New England Journal of Medicine* 337 (2 October 1997): 997–99.

Cystic Fibrosis and Gene Therapy

Enthusiasm for gene therapy in CF patients ran high in the 1990s, even though it was clear that gene therapy would not relieve all the symptoms of the disease. But the grand hope of a cure began to falter in the late 1990s, when gene therapy experiments produced severe side effects in subjects. And the venture suffered a devastating setback when Jesse Gelsinger—a young man with another disorder, OTC (ornithine transcarbamoylase) deficiency—died during a gene therapy experiment.

"I don't think chloride regulation is the sole defect, and I'm not sure it's the primary pathology, . . . [there is more to CF] than a failure to clear lung mucus."
—Richard Boucher, CF researcher, 1990

"Twenty years from now, gene therapy will have revolutionized the practice of medicine. Virtually every disease will have gene therapy as one of its treatments."
—W. French Anderson, gene therapy pioneer, 1996

"The new CF research shows that the [gene therapy] strategy works for an ever-increasing list of disorders where a defective gene is responsible . . . It gives credence to the idea that gene therapy will find a significant place in the therapeutic armamentarium."
—Francis Collins, director of the National Human Genome
    Research Institute and co-discoverer of the CF gene, 1990

"To think we're going to cure cystic fibrosis in a year is naïve, I'm not discouraged but this is going to take time and people shouldn't have unrealistic expectations."
—Ron Crystal, CF researcher, 1993

"They were going to inform me of everything they discovered . . . They were going to make me part of their team . . . [But they] were blinded by all the money, the prestige that was going to be attained by getting this to work, and willing to take risks with innocent people who didn't have the knowledge they need to know to be able to participate properly in this."
—Paul Gelsinger, father of Jesse Gelsinger, 2002

the enthusiasm for gene therapy shared much with the high expectations for heart-lung transplantation and other interventions. It represented dramatic new hope. But most important, the rise of gene therapy reflected a new kind of entrepreneurism. Over time, the gene therapy phenomenon reflected the growing influence of financial speculation and venture capital in clinical research.

As early as November 1985, the business media was reporting favorably on the financial promise of gene therapy targeted at particular populations. Noting that the age of "gene doctors" seemed to be upon us, *Business Week* magazine ran a cover story on the emergence of these physicians of the future—a group on the verge of "erasing nature's mistakes" and "curing life's cruelest diseases."[89] And when the *New York Times* headlines in October 1995 announced, "Genetic Marker for Cystic Fibrosis Reported Found," a prominent section heading—"Disease of Caucasians" —pointed to the expected beneficiaries, indicating that the population of those affected could be vast and yet also circumscribed by race.[90] Like lung transplantation, gene therapy emerged in the 1980s as a promising cottage research industry. But unlike HLT, which was developed in academic surgical units, the prospects for gene therapy would depend on larger sources of financing. From a very early date, gene therapy was also presented to the public as the object of a race among scientists and industry, the aim of that race being new kinds of treatments that "won't reach hospitals for years." But, it was claimed, this was an international race in which "the first experiments on humans are near."[91] These unabashedly speculative reports highlighted the enormous funding needs and capital potential of such experiments. Yet by 1990 the so-called gene doctors had actually achieved little beyond identifying CF genes.

From the beginning of the gene therapy enterprise, researchers promised exciting breakthroughs for patients with inherited disorders like cystic fibrosis, sickle cell disease, and hemophilia. But scientists would have to devise and test truly novel methods for introducing foreign genetic material into the body, preventing its rejection, and ensuring its safe functioning. Gene therapy gave rise to new kinds of research trials, for transferring genetic material was not quite the same as testing a new drug. In the 1970s and early 1980s, public and professional discussions usually fixated on a new drug only *after* it had passed through clinical trials and won approval for use. Nor was it equivalent to testing a new surgical procedure, even though gene therapy styled itself as more akin to surgical innovation (indeed, an early metaphor was "gene surgery"). There was no clear parallel between gene therapy and other modes of therapeutic innovation. In gene therapy, clinical research operated in this gray zone between drug testing and surgical innovation—and this, in part, gave the enterprise its revolutionary aura.[92] Even as they organized their experiments, researchers were also forming start-up companies, raising funds for these innovative therapies and seeking a market for them. The new gene doctors, then, blurred the distinctions between scientist and salesman, surgical pioneer and drug innovator, playing a role not just in developing new drugs and techniques but in testing them and in promoting them as well.

If the technique existed in an uncharted gray zone, so too did the researchers who mixed scientific investigation with the pursuit of profit. The new gene doctors were simultaneously researchers and entrepreneurs, conducting their clinical trials with profits in mind, acquiring stock in the enterprises they developed, or taking shares in the companies whose products their studies were evaluating. News articles relentlessly documented their efforts to correct the genetic abnormality, never allowing readers to lose sight of the fact that CF was "the most common lethal disease among white people, striking an estimated 30,000 Americans."[93] Such references to race and to the large potential population of CF patients conveyed to investors the scope of the problem and the symbolic import of the gene therapy venture. Building on these images, the gene doctors stoked ever-higher public expectations.

Enthusiasm for a gene-therapy cure for cystic fibrosis peaked in the early 1990s, when testing of a new gene delivery technique appeared imminent.[94] In 1993 the pulmonary specialist Ronald Crystal began the first experiment at the National Heart, Lung, and Blood Institute, using an adenovirus (a cold virus) as a vector to deliver genetic material to the lungs of a person with CF, "fulfilling hopes that had gathered locomotive force in the past several months," according to the New York Times. The study (one of three approved experiments) involved a twenty-three-year-old man with CF who, in the words of the newspaper, inhaled a cold virus that had been altered to "enclose a healthy copy of the cystic fibrosis gene the patient lacked." According to the theory, the gene in the virus, if taken up into the DNA of the lung tissue and expressed there, could possibly alter the impaired chloride transport in the lung cells of the patient. Although the article described the subject as a "patient" and was replete with references to "breakthroughs," "firsts," and "milestones," in reality the study intended to test not a treatment but rather a narrow yet crucial component of the theory: the efficacy of the gene transfer process. Amid the grandiose verbiage about "breakthroughs," this article acknowledged that "the man . . . is not likely to benefit clinically from the initial treatment, but will help scientists determine if the method has a chance of working and how long its effects last."[95] It was not uncommon for news media to create the mistaken impression that clinical studies to test the narrow problem of gene expression were a form of treatment. Newsweek, for example, casually announced that researchers were "learning to replace a faulty gene" and that Crystal planned to "treat" nine other adults with adenovirus, using gradually increasing doses.[96]

At the start of Crystal's experiments, researchers themselves spoke of gene therapy as an impending cure, although some remained cautious about the true implications for patients.[97] As physician Bonnie Ramsey stated with certainty and in typically grandiose terms, "In the next decade, we are going to see a revolution in treatment for this disease. We can really, truly think about a cure." Yet some parents, those who had learned firsthand about the pros and cons of antibiotics and lung transplants, were more cautiously optimistic. As one pointed out, "We're fully aware that whatever they come up with may not be in time for our daughter." The realities of lung deterioration also raised questions about the precise benefits gene therapy could and could not deliver. Could it, for example, repair already damaged lung tissue? Not likely. Would it be as useful in older CF patients as in younger ones? Probably not, noted one observer, since "most patients past puberty have already suffered too much lung damage to be saved by even the most sophisticated therapies."[98]

As gene therapy emerged into the trial phase, the race to serve this growing cohort of patients and to relieve their pain was moving forward rapidly, partly because the economic opportunities were so great. Biotechnology firms had already invested large sums in the hunt for novel CF drugs. In March 1993 Genentech, Inc., requested permission from the FDA to market a cystic fibrosis drug called DNase that had been shown in clinical trials to reduce respiratory infections and improve breathing. *Business Week* proclaimed, "A star drug is born."[99] Another article commented that "Genentech's stock rose 50 cents a share" after the announcement.[100] A third pointed out that DNase, marketed under the brand name Pulmozyme, was only one player in a "$600 million dollar horse race" in which many companies, from small start-ups to biotechnology giants, were trying "to capture the potentially lucrative gene therapy market." Leading the pack was Ron Crystal, identified as "co-founder of gene therapy start-up Gen-Vec in Rockville, Maryland," with $17 million of capital support from Genentech and facilities presumably in close proximity to his offices at the National Heart, Lung, and Blood Institute.[101]

In late 1993 Crystal's venture, and along with it gene therapy's prospects, hit a serious snag when his third "patient" developed a number of troubling symptoms: lung inflammation, a drop in oxygen levels in the blood, and evidence of pulmonary damage. These events exposed the enormous differences between, on one hand, large-scale clinical trials, with large numbers of subjects, drugs well-vetted for safety, and researchers "blinded" so that their biases would not shape the results, and, on the other hand, studies like Crystal's involving a handful of individuals, unproven agents and procedures, and researchers fully conscious of the financial import of their findings. When the troubling symptoms arose, Crystal rushed to defend his venture, speculating that this "patient" may have been "idiosyncratic." At the same time he acknowledged that these events could plausibly suggest that the "upper limits" of adenovirus therapy had been reached. Crystal backed away from broad claims of curing CF, and the reporter remarked that the incident underscored "the difficulties of turning a highly experimental therapy into a workaday clinical method." The setback prompted a renewed focus on the hypothesis-testing features of what were now termed early-stage trials, "simply designed to explore questions of safety, to determine whether the gene switches on once the adenovirus has infected lung cells and to learn how long the effect lasts." [102] Signs that adenovirsues caused lower oxygen levels, inflammation, and possibly lung damage as well as other side effects ultimately forced Crystal and several other scientists to revise the expectations of the early 1990s and to stress the experimental character of their gene therapy research. Some advocates even suggested that the wisdom of the adenovirus approach itself needed to be reevaluated.

Unmitigated optimism gave way to cautious hope as the gene therapy enterprise came more clearly into focus as "experimental." Extensive discussions of gene therapy's limitations would follow. "Despite their enthusiasm," noted one survey in a 1994 issue of *Discover*, "researchers know there are potential drawbacks." [103] Another 1995 survey of the field in *Science* commented, "Right from the start, gene therapists have recognized that their central challenge would be to find safe vectors capable of transporting genes efficiently into target cells — and getting the cells to express the genes once they are inserted." [104] Notably, observers also began to acknowledge that the procedure (even if successful) was unlikely to be a one-time fix; rather, the method would probably involve frequent treatments, since "lung epithelial cells are shed about every two or three months . . . [and] the new genes' efficacy seems to last only a few weeks."[105] Such speculation was premature in 1994, for everyone now acknowledged that key problems of safety and efficacy remained. One problem, which had severe implications for gene therapy's efficacy, was the inflammation caused by the immune system's response to the adenovirus. Simply stated, the virus looked "like a foreign invader to the immune system, so after repeated exposures, a patient's immune system could learn to drive off the virus before it delivers its load."[106] Another limitation, according to researcher Richard Boucher, was that gene therapy researchers were caught in a dilemma about dosage. "When administered at low concentrations [the adenovirus] is ineffective . . . at high doses, however, it appears to cause acute inflammation."[107] To be sure, optimism continued, but it was a more cautious "experimental" optimism. Promoters of the gene therapy enterprise continued to believe that CF was the ideal target disease to prove the worth of the adenovirus approach to gene therapy; it was, as one source noted, "just the opponent gene therapy has been looking for." Optimism remained a crucial force in sustaining the flow of venture capital for the research enterprise, and entrepreneurs continued to see the disease as an opportunity for demonstrating the promise of their agenda.[108]

To be sure, there was money to be made in day-to-day cystic fibrosis care, but gene therapy seemed to be a far more lucrative prospect because of the large, relatively privileged market of patients and the frustrations of patients, families, and doctors with the therapeutic status quo. *Science* magazine's 1995 survey provided an overview of the "hundreds of millions of dollars at stake." Many businesses pressed forward in the race for gene therapy, even as researchers now made more cautious claims. As the *Science* article put it, "Academic researchers are still grappling with fundamental issues in gene therapy. But industry leaders and their financial agents are gung-ho."[109] Such tensions were, of course, not confined to gene therapy and CF, for throughout the 1980s and 1990s the close ties between private enterprise and university research stirred debate about the influence of money on objectivity and the ethics of these research arrangements.[110] James Wilson, director of the Institute for Gene Therapy at the University of Pennsylvania and one of gene therapy's early proponents, acknowledged that "commercial pressure may . . . account for some of the hype surrounding developments in gene therapy . . . If you're the leader of a gene-therapy company, you try to put as positive a spin as you can on every step of the research process . . . because you have to create promise out of what you have—that's your value."[111]

Frank assessments like this one made clear that researchers like Ron Crystal were a troubling modern hybrid: the researcher/entrepreneur. The company Crystal had co-founded, GenVec, Inc., with $20 million in capital, was one of fourteen companies that had invested hundreds of millions of dollars in the grand venture.[112] In the minds of many cystic fibrosis researchers, such ventures were not a problem but a solution. Many patients, family members, and policy makers agreed. When the U.S. Senate Committee on Small Business held hearings in 1994 on "research on childhood diseases by entrepreneurs," speakers testified that "gene therapy holds the promise of a cure for CF."[113] In their view, gene therapy was destined to "transform medicine."[114] But where some saw promise, breakthrough, and profit, others perceived an increasingly troubled enterprise. At the heart of the problem was a potentially dangerous vehicle (the adenovirus) and an increasingly problematic relationship among clinician-researchers, CF patients and their families, entrepreneurial venture capital, and the biotechnology market.

Cystic fibrosis gene therapy was not going as planned, and the real prospect emerged that the disease and the technique might not be made for one another after all. By the mid-1990s, some researchers had begun to discuss explicitly how faith in gene therapy had perpetuated a narrow view of CF as a lung disease, thereby obscuring the complex biological character of the disease and enormous variations in how individual patients experienced the disease.[115] Richard Boucher acknowledged as early as 1990, "I don't think chloride regulation is the sole defect, and I'm not sure it's the primary pathology," suggesting that there was more to CF "than a failure to clear lung mucus."[116] The promise of gene therapy continued to captivate the business world and reporters, one of whom called it "bottling the stuff of dreams."[117] But researchers and biotech companies increasingly acknowledged the problems with the adenovirus model and with gene therapy's focus on cystic fibrosis. Following a series of disappointing setbacks, Crystal commented in 1998 that whereas CF required regular expression from the introduced gene, by contrast "for certain cancers and cardiovascular disease, you don't need expression forever." Accordingly, the company he founded, GenVec, was now "concentrating on gene therapy for cardiovascular disease." Similarly, after eight unsuccessful gene therapy trials for CF, the chief scientific officer at Genzyme Corporation announced, "Maybe the quickest route to solving cystic fibrosis is to take a detour."[118] The vast enterprise had apparently moved on, to make promises (and overpromises) to other patients, families, and disease constituencies. The gene therapy train was headed off in new, more promising and potentially profitable directions, leaving CF patients at the station.[119]

Viewed in retrospect, the enthusiasm surrounding gene therapy for cystic fibrosis was close kin with the dot-com bubble of the 1990s.[120] Mirroring the wave of heavy investment in computer and Internet-related companies, venture capital investment in gene therapy poured vast sums into companies seeking breakthrough therapies for potentially lucrative markets of patients. Pharmaceutical companies threw their support behind pioneering research scientists at the helm of smaller start-up ventures. In those heady days many clinical research entrepreneurs became speculators and made large personal investments in this part of the biotech boom—rewriting old rules about objectivity and research ethics. For many, gene therapy was the holy grail of biomedical research. Gene therapy offered to bring the CF patient something fundamentally different from antibacterial therapy, comprehensive management, or lung transplantation: gene therapy promised cure. Yet this promise was a product of the broader speculative fervor surrounding the technology-based stock market, and every observer knew that it far exceeded any demonstrated efficacy. Yet almost all of the main players also believed that this was a secure investment in the future of both medicine and cystic fibrosis care.

INVESTMENT IN BAD DREAMS:
THE DEATH OF JESSE GELSINGER

How did the dream of genetic medicine and efforts to bring genetic therapies to the medical marketplace exploit ideas of identity, partnership, risk taking, and breakthrough medicine? By the late 1990s the gene therapy campaign had moved away from cystic fibrosis to other research terrain, to other diseases—some of them more obscure than CF and others better known. In the wake of problems with gene therapy for cystic fibrosis, the University of Pennsylvania researchers led by James Wilson had abandoned CF as their model disease, deciding instead to take up a new disorder called ornithine transcarbamoylase deficiency and to use another modified adenovirus. This time they hoped for smoother sailing toward a cure. But the ensuing controversy would reveal even more about the enterprise. In 1999 the dream of an easy cure suffered another stunning setback: the sudden death of an eighteen-year-old man named Jesse Gelsinger who was participating in a gene therapy experiment at Penn. The Gelsinger case quickly turned the spotlight away from the "promising miracle" of genetic transformation and focused it on the industry itself—on how it sold its claims and how such an industry should be regulated.

Although the Gelsinger case does not concern cystic fibrosis per se, it focused the microscope on the scientists themselves and drew public attention to how boosters of gene therapy sold exalted promises of genetic transformation to patients, their families, and the public, and how the hype played upon people's broader faith in risk taking and in the power of the marketplace to improve their lives. A close look at the case allows us to draw some final conclusions about the selling of the dream of genetic transformation, to scrutinize those who bought into the dream, and to explore the powerful and widely shared assumptions about the marketplace that sustained the appeal of this dream for many mainstream Americans — if only for a limited time.

On 17 September 1999, eighteen-year-old Jesse Gelsinger died after developing complications resulting from his participation in a gene transfer experiment at the University of Pennsylvania. Although the cause of his death would be disputed for some time to come, first indications suggested that his body had experienced an acute immune response to the adenovirus that researchers were using to try to transfer a healthy, functioning gene into Jesse's impaired liver. Jesse had been a lifelong sufferer of the rare disorder ornithine transcarbamoylase (OTC) deficiency, a metabolic disease that impaired his liver's ability to rid itself of ammonia.[121] His death had immediate implications for both gene therapy research and cystic fibrosis research, for it suggested that some of the very features that had made CF and OTC appealing test cases for gene therapy also made patients vulnerable as research subjects. As *New York Times* journalist Sheryl Gay Stolberg put it, "Every realm of medicine has its defining moment, often with a face attached. Polio had Jonas Salk. In vitro fertilization had Louise Brown, the world's first test tube baby. Transplant surgery had Barney Clark, the Seattle dentist with the artificial heart. AIDS had Magic Johnson. And now gene therapy has Jesse Gelsinger."[122]

Like many of the cystic fibrosis patients who embraced gene therapy in the 1990s, Jesse Gelsinger was willing to take risks. He was at a crossroads with regard to his disease and his life. He had been lucky enough to survive infancy and childhood with his disorder and to arrive at a point where he could make critical decisions for himself about the course of his therapy. Immediately after his eighteenth birthday—indeed, on the very day he ceased to be a minor—Jesse flew to Philadelphia from his home in Tucson, Arizona, to begin experimental gene therapy with a team of researchers led by James Wilson. Only recently had the Penn researchers turned away from CF gene therapy experiments, hoping that OTC would prove to be a more malleable target disease. The Penn research team had devised a protocol for testing an adenovirus that had been modified to carry a functional OTC gene into the impaired livers of nineteen patients, Jesse among them. Like CF researcher Ron Crystal a few years earlier, the Penn researchers believed that their modified adenovirus would safely express detectable levels of OTC in human patients deficient in the enzyme. Classified by the FDA as a phase I clinical trial, the experiment was designed to test the safety of the technique, including levels of toxicity, and promised no therapeutic benefit to Jesse or the other OTC-deficient patients participating in the experiment. A crucial lesson had been learned from the CF studies of previous years: Wilson's team did not appear to glorify or oversell the therapeutic possibilities.

Jesse, the youngest patient in the trial, was chosen to receive the highest dose of adenovirus, which, researchers explained, would likely produce flulike symptoms. Penn researchers made it clear to Jesse and his father, Paul—both of whom signed informed-consent forms—that any improvements in his condition that might possibly stem from the experiment would not last and that the experiment entailed several kinds of risk. A day of surgery was necessary to administer the virus; the expected flulike symptoms would warrant an overnight stay in the hospital; and there were risks posed by the liver biopsy that would be required to ascertain if Jesse's liver was expressing OTC by way of the genetically modified virus. The researchers also mentioned risks of bleeding, blood clots, hepatitis, liver failure, and other postsurgical complications.[123] Paul Gelsinger chose not to make the trip to Philadelphia with his son because, as he understood it, the most dangerous part of the procedure was the liver biopsy that would follow the injection of the adenovirus by a few days. Asked later about the adenovirus, Paul recalled believing that "there was no great risk there, that [the Penn researchers] hadn't seen any really bad side effects, that there was just flu-like symptoms . . . The way they described it, this thing looked so safe. Jesse was going to get the flu."[124]

By the late 1990s, of course, researchers knew well that the body's response to the gene therapy vector—inflammation, fever, and "the flu"—constituted a significant challenge to patients, but few were prepared for what the vector appeared to provoke in Jesse Gelsinger's body. The word flu conveyed the concern in terms that families could understand, but as the Gelsingers would soon learn, it did not accurately describe the body's physiological response. While no one could immediately ascertain what caused Jesse's death, his health deteriorated rapidly on 13 September in the hours following the injection of the adenovirus. A severe immune response led to what the Penn doctors initially described as "multiple organ failure."[125] Jesse's ammonia levels became dangerously elevated. By the next morning, other symptoms suggested that his red blood cells were breaking down faster than his liver could metabolize them.[126] As ammonia levels in Jesse's blood rose, coma, lung failure, and brain death followed. After four days and a series of desperate efforts to combat these catastrophic symptoms, the doctors finally advised the Gelsinger family to remove Jesse from life support. The trial was immediately halted.[127]

Over the following year, Paul Gelsinger's relationship with the Penn researcher gradually deteriorated, and the unfolding story became a lens through which the entire gene therapy enterprise, with its hype and inflated promises, was scrutinized. As the Penn researchers set out to investigate the events leading to Jesse's death, they shared news of their findings with the distraught father every step of the way. Initially he harbored no enmity toward the researchers, and he defended Jesse's doctors, telling reporters, "They are good people. Their intent was pure."[128]

By September 2000, however, Paul Gelsinger's view of the

events had changed as he learned more about the financial interests of the researchers. A year after his son's death, Paul concluded that the Penn research team had fraudulently and negli-
gently recruited Jesse into their clinical trials, and he filed a suit
against James Wilson and three other doctors on the team.[129] After
a tumultuous year spent participating in investigations into Jesse's
death and into the claims of the gene therapy industry, Paul Gelsinger stated, "They were going to inform me of everything they
discovered . . . They were going to make me part of their team
. . . [But they] were blinded by all the money, the prestige that was
going to be attained by getting this to work, and willing to take
risks with innocent people who didn't have the knowledge they
need to know to be able to participate properly in this."[130] Jesse's
family—along with major regulators, peer institutions, and other
scientists—concluded that the "partnership" between Jesse and
his doctors had been little more than an elaborate fiction. The
FDA had taken the lead in investigating whether the Penn researchers had hoodwinked the agency and other regulatory bodies
into approving the experiments by not disclosing the true risks
involved.[131] After its own reassessment, the FDA chastised Wilson and his colleagues for playing down previously noted warning
signs; for example, they had failed to report serious side effects
in two of the subjects who had been successfully "treated" before
Gelsinger.

What most outraged FDA investigators, Paul Gelsinger, and
others was the specter of the profit motive skewing scientific judgment.[132] This topic had been a source of concern to some critics
for years. But the Gelsinger investigation put a human face to this
story of money and science, thus transforming the moral terrain
around gene therapy. The FDA's investigation revealed that James
Wilson had founded a company that held the rights to any successful treatments using the adenovirus, and investigators found
this to be a significant conflict of interest that clouded Wilson's
assessment of risks and benefits. In these and many other ways,
the FDA argued, the integrity of the research process had been

compromised. Not surprisingly, the investigators also found that material posted on the Penn website to recruit volunteer subjects contained misleadingly optimistic language about the benefits potentially stemming from the experiment.[133] The Gelsinger scandal damaged the careers of some of the most prominent gene therapy entrepreneurs of the 1990s, including James Wilson (who nevertheless earned $13.5 million when his company was sold to Targeted Genetics Corp. of Seattle in 2000).[134] From this point forward, the claims of those conducting experimental gene therapy were subjected to greater scrutiny. Clinical trials halted under a heavy cloud of suspicion.[135]

Some Americans felt betrayed. Like Paul Gelsinger, they had developed a strong sense of trust that gene therapy research was a true partnership between scientist and subject. But both they and Gelsinger began to learn of the Penn team's errors and tactical omissions from a series of public meetings held at the NIH in December 1999. To be sure, the gene therapists had many defenders at these hearings. When James Wilson and the Penn researchers denied the allegations of impropriety, supporters rallied to their side.[136] Parents of critically ill children, for example, testified about the critical need to continue gene therapy research despite the tragedy of Jesse's death. For them, the possibilities of a dramatic cure through gene therapy still lingered in the air. However, several researchers admitted their failure to disclose adverse side effects and other events to the FDA and NIH, and they offered heartfelt apologies.[137] At first, Paul Gelsinger supported of the Penn researchers. But as he listened to their blunt admissions that there was "no significant statistical data" showing benefit to patients exposed to adenovirus, he became convinced, as he put it later, that "I had been misled."[138] And as in the case of Ronald Crystal and cystic fibrosis gene therapy, retrospective investigations disclosed the existence of previously unreported deaths—deaths that at the time were attributed to the patients' underlying disease but could now be seen as linked to the effects of gene therapy itself.[139] The popular media now knew that Jesse Gelsinger was not the sole casualty of the genetics revolution, and exposés on "death at the hands of science" undermined faith in the partnership between researchers and their subjects.[140]

The Gelsinger case allowed observers to see clearly the inner workings of the culture of hype and promise that shaped the dream of gene therapy for cystic fibrosis in the 1980s and 1990s. Investigations afterward also made clear that the deregulatory impulse of the era was a major, if invisible, actor in the drama. Reagan- and Bush-era zeal for private enterprise and deregulation had shifted the balance between the public and private sectors, systematically undermining the government's regulatory role in many arenas. The trend continued under the Clinton administration. In a *New York Times* article reassessing the Gelsinger case, Sheryl Gay Stolberg linked the episode to the history of a little-known regulatory body, the Recombinant DNA Advisory Committee (RAC), and explained how its loss of regulatory authority over the gene therapy enterprise in 1995 precipitated the tragedy.[141]

Two powerful forces were driving the deregulatory impulse and nurturing Americans' cultural investments in the dream of gene therapy. The first was the biotechnology and pharmaceutical industry itself, which was intent on reducing barriers to the approval and marketing of new products; the industry had little tolerance for those who held back innovation out of concern for protecting vulnerable patients.[142] The second force was the patient advocacy movement — groups of patient activists desperate for faster access to experimental drugs. A case in point would be the AIDS activists of the 1980s who successfully pressured the FDA to "fast-track" its approval process.[143] Of particular concern for gene therapy researchers was the perception that RAC oversight of gene therapy trials was unnecessarily duplicative. In the end, the risk-taking patients and the innovators found common cause in the ideology of gene therapy, and regulators stood back and waited for events to unfold. Behind the gene therapy revolution lay a political revolution.[144]

The enormous optimism surrounding gene therapy in the

1990s was deeply ideological, entangled with American political, business, and mainstream cultural values. Despite the warnings heard in the 1980s about the mingling of business and scientific interests, the exploitation of research subjects, and the risks (known and unknown) of genetic experimentation, the genetics revolution would not wait. The champions of gene therapy dismissed the objections as nay-saying and negativism in the face of the can-do spirit. Advocates claimed that success would ultimately allay all these concerns. Research subjects were neither guinea pigs nor a means toward business profit but true partners in a grand pursuit, sharing equally in the fruits of discovery. But with the death of Jesse Gelsinger, such expressions of hope gave way to accusations about the exploitation of trust and the overselling of a dream. And the once-invisible ideological components of the dream could now (at least for a short time) be visualized.

"BASICALLY, IT'S A WHITE DISEASE": CYSTIC FIBROSIS AND MYTHS OF RACE

Cystic fibrosis was surrounded by many myths, many of which remained invisible and unchallenged, and all of which needed to be constantly nurtured by advocates. One of them was the myth of imminent breakthrough, the promise that the peaks of success would grow ever higher, that imperfect technologies were perfectible, and that dying patients could be made well again. Researchers' and patients' faith in this myth and their quick embrace of gene therapy cannot be separated from their sense that CF care had indeed reached a frustrating plateau. This idea was so central to the thinking of many doctors, families, and patients that it could be exploited by anyone who had something better to sell, something more clear-cut and definitive. The idea of gene therapy for cystic fibrosis filled an emotional need, but in the end it was a marketing myth, revealing more about the business culture and mainstream ideologies of the 1990s than about the actual potential of genetic technology. Moreover, the very logic of gene therapy depended upon a radical oversimplification of a complex, multi-dimensional disorder.

A powerful history of trust, partnership, and belief in innovative treatments took an unfortunate turn in the gene therapy chapter of the cystic fibrosis story. During the post–World War II decades, CF patients had grown into adolescence and young adulthood dependent on antibiotics and in close relationships with doctors and research scientists (and to some extent with pharmaceutical companies). Cystic fibrosis care in the home had long been portrayed as an extension of lifesaving comprehensive care in the hospital, and the partnership between parents and doctors as the central element in progress toward a cure. The home life of the child with CF stood in stark contrast to that of the child with Tay-Sachs disease, doomed from the start to an inevitable decline. But the very progress that had been achieved in CF had become a source of frustration. By the 1980s, life expectancy for CF patients had increased dramatically (from 3–5 years to 30–35 years), and with this transformation came expectations for better care. Of course the benefits were not evenly spread; at least one study found that "medically indigent patients form a subgroup whose mortality and morbidity are significantly worse than those of the population of CF patients as a whole."[145] On the whole, however, patients' improving fortunes (tinged as they were with frustration) made it easy for many of them to trust surgeons in the 1980s who championed heart-lung transplants, or genetic researchers in the 1990s who made increasingly grand promises about gene therapy.

There was, of course, another myth about cystic fibrosis making the rounds in the 1990s: the notion that all "white people," all majority Americans who identified as such, had a stake in CF and the genetic enterprise. Proponents of genetic research and gene therapy for cystic fibrosis invoked the idea of CF as a "Caucasian disease" not to raise dollars but to communicate the broad implications of their work. For example, with the discovery of the DF508 mutation responsible for nearly two-thirds of CF cases, many researchers believed that to trace the prevalence of this mutation around the world was to track European identity itself. But what they discovered was puzzling, for the pattern of the DF508 mutation did not conform to the popular stereotype of cystic fibrosis as a disease among white people of Northern European ancestry. Prevalence varied across Europe, with higher rates reported, for example, in places like Jordan and Ireland than in most parts of France and Northern Europe. As writings on the DF508 gene mutation for cystic fibrosis make clear, the myth of the disease's whiteness needed to be constantly nurtured, refined, and shored up in light of new research findings suggesting a more complex demographic profile.

In the 1970s, Giulio Barbero and other researchers who drew attention to cystic fibrosis had stressed its panethnic identity, its reach across many groups, and its incidence among black as well as white Americans, in order to encourage a broader cultural investment in the disease; but increasingly in the 1980s, researchers and the mass media signaled to their readers that CF should be understood as a white person's disorder. It was, in the words of one observer, the "white version of sickle cell disease," a remark implying a bid for the same kind of attention being given to other ethnic maladies like Tay-Sachs and sickle cell disease. "Basically, it's a white disease," pronounced Frank Deford in a 1986 *Washington Post* interview about his biography of his daughter Alex.[146] A few years earlier, another *Washington Post* article made the link to whiteness more explicit, noting that an avowedly racist and antisemitic organization known as the National Socialist White People's Party had taken up the disease as one of its causes, raising "funds to support research in cystic fibrosis and other disease that [the party's leader] asserted primarily strike people of Northern European ancestry."[147]

This association of whiteness and cystic fibrosis with the new capital-intensive gene therapy venture is no coincidence. To highlight the "whiteness" of cystic fibrosis was, in a sense, to attempt to sell a concept, to suggest that CF gene therapy had a vast market, to rally investors and patient constituencies to the idea. Genetics entrepreneurs had particular markets in mind, in much the same way that pharmaceutical companies targeted drugs to particular consumer groups. CF's "whiteness" projected clearly who the beneficiaries of gene therapy would be—the majority of Americans—just as legislative attention to sickle cell disease years earlier had communicated a vision of how resources would be distributed to African Americans.

The race problem in cystic fibrosis is a complicated one. In France, where high rates of CF have been found in the northwestern region of Brittany (which some characterize as a "Celtic" region), the "white" or "European" nature of the disease can have little meaning.[148] But in America, whiteness is an extremely flexible and potent concept. Two hundred years ago it was quite specific, denoting people of Anglo-Saxon heritage. It later expanded to subsume waves of ethnic immigrants once labeled "colored," from Irish to Jewish to Italians and other Europeans. For these groups, the idea of "whiteness" has come to signify broader processes of acculturation to an American ideal, the giving up of specific Old World identities in exchange for a more secure place in American society. It has also come to mean identifying with an American majority culture and its ideals of capital accumulation, middle-class values, and (increasingly in the 1980s and 1990s), faith in the marketplace.

Even if the idea would have meant little in a nation like France, the link between cystic fibrosis and whiteness seemed compelling in the American mind-set of the 1990s. Most stories about the disease and the possibilities of gene therapies reinforced that this disease was a "white" or "Caucasian" concern. A 1994 *Washington Post* story noted, for example, that "one in 20 Caucasians harbors a mutated CFTR gene."[149] It was common to read, as the *Atlanta Journal and Constitution* noted in 1998, that CF was "the most common fatal inherited disease among Caucasians."[150] It was not merely a threat to white Americans but a global challenge. As a *New York Times* article in 2003 noted, CF was "the most common life-shortening genetic disease among Caucasians worldwide."[151]

Amid the focus on cystic fibrosis as an experience with which white Americans might identify regardless of their ethnic background, some media did highlight the panethnic profile. A 1995 *Minnesota Star Tribune* article, for example, made the usual observation that CF was "one of the most common inherited disorders of Caucasians," occurring in 1 of every 2,500 live births, but also noted that CF occurred in 1 of every 17,000 births among African Americans and was rare among Asians and Native Americans.[152]

These reports would be received differently in their different locales—New York City, Atlanta, Minneapolis, Washington, D.C.—but they all suggested that this story of genetic transformation was to some extent a story about and for whites. The very notion of *white people* was, of course, a convenient amalgam, a powerful symbolic reference group for all Americans, whether they belonged to that group or not. The term *white* collapsed a wide range of groups with diverse heritages—from Irish to Italians, from Jews to Northern and Southern Europeans, from English to Germans and Eastern Europeans—into a single category, encouraging them to identify with one another. *White* operated in much the same way that *people of color* or *black* did: to create a unified perspective and set of cultural investments.

If Tay-Sachs disease had been etched into the national psyche as a Jewish genetic disease and sickle cell disease had been cultivated for twenty years as an index of the black experience, cystic fibrosis was a story about genes, suffering, faith, and genetic transformation as part of the white experience in America. Indeed, what made the story particularly American was that the very idea of its whiteness remained unanalyzed. "Whiteness" signified the erasure of particular ethnic identities and cultural heritages and the imparting of a new set of ideas about common values and commitments, common histories, and common suffering. Alongside this racial ethos ran another one that was also about transformation: faith in the ability of business and medicine to deliver on the promise of innovation, to make sick people better by way of radical if risky measures. As we shall see in the next chapter, such ideologies of transformation were not universally embraced. A very different ethos defined how physicians, scientists, families, and patients struggled with the dream of genetic medicine in sickle cell disease.

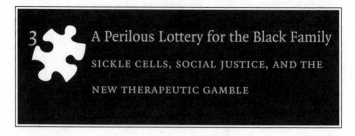

Patients with sickle cell disease (SCD) and their physicians have often responded skeptically to grand claims about therapeutic breakthroughs. Hugh Chaplin, a specialist in hematology, put it this way: "These patients are on a roller coaster ride of unrealistic expectations and heartbreak as one announced 'breakthrough' after another has failed to materialize." In a 2003 book dedicated to his longtime patient Lenabell McClelland, Chaplin asked, "Is there anyone to blame for this?" Were journalists and pharmaceutical companies responsible? Or were medical researchers and patients themselves engaging in "premature 'hype'"? In the end, Chaplin concluded, the roller-coaster ride was not the fault of any particular group, yet the pattern remained clear and puzzling. "The story turns up in a national newspaper or on a television news broadcast," he said. "Later it turns out that enthusiasm for this 'breakthrough' is not justified and nothing further is heard about the drug."[1] That an established hematologist voiced such concerns indicates that the particular sensibilities surrounding sickle cell disease were perhaps radically different from those surrounding cystic fibrosis (CF) and Tay-Sachs disease (TSD).

For nearly a century, and in varying ways, sickle cell disease has been characterized in the United States as a "black disease." As a malady especially prevalent in African-American families, it has been shadowed by a politics of mistrust. In recent years this mistrust has often been attributed to the "legacy of Tuskegee" and past histories of racial discrimination in medical care.[2] In the particular history of SCD, however, patients' experiences with the health care system and with therapies shaped their expectations and sensibilities.

Indeed, the race question in sickle cell disease has a complex history, in which the politics of race has played the critical role while the biology of race has been an elusive shadow. Scientists in the 1950s and 1960s saw the disease as an African inheritance, and they theorized that sickle cell carriers (the heterozygote parents of patients) possessed a beneficial resistance to *falciparum* malaria, and thus had a survival advantage over other people in the areas of Africa where malaria was prevalent. Over centuries the heterozygote advantage grew in these regions, but so too did the likelihood of two such people having children together and giving birth to a child with sickle cell disease. Scientists learned, however, that SCD was only one of a widely distributed number of similar hemoglobin disorders—a close cousin to thalassemia, for example, which was prevalent in the Mediterranean, in Greece and in Italy, where malaria also figured prominently. Thus region and malaria appeared to be crucial to the evolution of both SCD and thalassemia. Yet experts pondering SCD tended to see the disease as an index of fundamental biological race differences. By contrast, few would suggest that thalassemia's prevalence meant that Italians or Greeks were different biological races. The race question in SCD in America hinged, by and large, on political rather than scientific calculations.[3]

As a disease marked by recurring pain and suffering, SCD also emerged in the 1960s and 1970s as a powerful symbol of the African-American experience.[4] Into the 1980s and 1990s, and still today, everything about SCD has carried profound cultural meaning. From the pain, the infections, and the high mortality rates to the African inheritance and the roller coaster of unfulfilled therapeutic promises, every aspect of SCD in the United States speaks to the problem of "race" and the social condition of African Americans.

In the years when gene therapy was rising to prominence, promising imminent relief for patients with the "Caucasian" disease cystic fibrosis, and when "genetic matchmaking" was taking center stage in the fight against Tay-Sachs disease in Ultra-Orthodox Jewish communities, sickle cell patients too faced a complex set of promises and dilemmas. To read the popular and professional discussions of these genetic maladies is to see very different stories unfolding, for different cultural values were at stake in each community of suffering.[5] The diseases were microcosms of very different kinds of ethnic politics. In the case of CF, years of partnership between researchers and families, as well as significant resources for comprehensive care, had helped build a stable and effective system of care as well as a shared belief in the transformative power of innovative medicine. A culture of risk-taking and entrepreneurship animated this partnership. By the 1990s, many believed that "gene therapy" would push progress to an entirely new level, delivering the long-awaited cure for CF patients who were living longer and yet remained frustrated by their day-to-day challenges. In the case of Tay-Sachs disease, the story was not about faith in imminent cures. Rather, it was about innovative methods of preventing the birth of Tay-Sachs babies, about Jewish self-determination, and about the lengths to which a small minority community might go to safeguard its families and guard itself against a wide range of genetic diseases that were apparently established in their world.

The story of sickle cell disease from the 1950s into the 1990s, by contrast, followed a path characterized by incremental progress, recurring promises of breakthrough cures, and highly publicized disappointments. In contrast to the cystic fibrosis story, a reliable system of comprehensive care still eluded many sickle cell patients. Many observers, like Chaplin, had seen enormous advances over the years, yet they also believed that basic services were needed and that the promise of cure was overly simplistic. Patients and researchers alike always held out hope for therapeutic progress. But over the decades the exalted faith and hype regarding imminent cures became muted as efforts to cure SCD confronted a series of troublesome social realities, such as access to basic health care.

The idea of risky high-tech innovations, in this context of deprivation, would spawn controversy. Indeed, by the 1990s innovation in SCD care had come to be seen as a dangerous game—a tricky act of balancing the promises of dramatic advances and the perils posed by extraordinary medical experiments against the difficulties of accessing standard medical care. In short, the cultural meaning of innovation was not the same as in the world of cystic fibrosis. Controversy swirled about the use of urea in the 1970s and appeared again two decades later in discussions of bone marrow transplantation. Against this historical backdrop, what did the revolution in genetic medicine promise to sickle cell patients and their families? What did it mean to pursue high-risk cures?

The roller-coaster ride of sickle cell therapeutics offers an object lesson about the politics of black identity in America. For some, the story that follows may highlight ironies of being black in modern America; for others, the story may point to the persistence of sometimes astonishingly racist attitudes in medicine and elsewhere; and for yet others, the story may evoke how black identity politics comes into play in every arena of American life, including the medical arena. A particular ethos surrounded questions of therapeutics in SCD. Whatever the meanings of its therapeutic history, the story of sickle cell disease draws attention to how the disease and innovative treatments for it intertwine with particular questions of justice and race in America.

In 1993, while people with cystic fibrosis looked forward to breakthrough improvements in care with the advent of gene therapy, sickle cell patients and their doctors viewed gene therapy with a strong sense of ambivalence. In SCD, it was not gene therapy but another innovation—bone marrow transplantation—that became a focal point of intense debates, taking on the same kind of cultural importance that gene therapy did in cystic fibrosis. The prospect of bone marrow transplantation raised similar issues for the SCD community as gene therapy raised in the CF community. Some saw the experimental method—transplanting new bone marrow cells into sick patients in order to produce normal red blood cells—as fulfilling the promise of a permanent cure. Yet it was also clear that bone marrow transplantation was a perilous lottery. The risks of the procedure ran very high, including the real possibility of death—anywhere between 10 and 30 percent mortality during the procedure. In the minds of many experts, these risks far outweighed the benefits and dictated that few patients or families should be offered the gamble at such bad odds.

The debate reflected competing perspectives on innovation within the sickle cell community. In the community of doctors and patients knowledgeable about SCD, there was a deeply ingrained, and historically shaped, ambivalence about dramatic claims of cure. This sensibility was, in a way, part of the cultural ethos of the disease, and it surfaced repeatedly in the history of SCD therapeutics, playing itself out whenever discussions turned to new therapies. Discussions of SCD therapeutics often became an occasion for imagining the black family and community and for reflecting on the health care system itself. In the case of SCD, then, as with the genetic diseases considered in earlier chapters, questions about therapeutics could never be easily separated from specific cultural debates about the people afflicted.

Although the story of sickle cell disease and bone marrow transplantation bears some resemblance to the history of cystic fibrosis and gene therapy, it also resembles the narrative of Tay-Sachs disease and the Dor Yeshorim in that experts, lay people, white Americans, and African Americans all had well-established ideas about black identity in relation to the disease. Unlike Ultra-Orthodox Jews who embraced genetic screening and counseling as a means of eradicating TSD, many African Americans were skeptical about genetic screening and counseling for SCD. For some of them, screening and prevention seemed to be part of a long history—beginning with slavery—of coercive reproductive practices and violations of their rights of self-determination by the white majority. In the early 1970s, many African Americans responded with suspicion to carrier testing for sickle cell disease. Revelations about the decades-long Tuskegee study of untreated syphilis in black men in Alabama merely accentuated these suspicions. In SCD's history, therefore, problems of historical experience, ethnic control, black identity, and the pursuit of social justice eclipsed arguments for breakthrough therapies.[6]

Such cultural factors as these help to explain why, in the 1990s, many researchers, patients, and doctors concerned with sickle cell disease felt a certain ambivalence about gene therapy and other innovations, even though gene therapy researchers and journalists frequently pointed to SCD as a likely beneficiary of the genetics revolution. In 1993, in the wake of a gene therapy trial on an infant with a severe immune deficiency disorder, one researcher promised that "if this procedure is found to be effective . . . it will open a door" so that "inherited disease like sickle cell anemia and hemophilia might be cured in newborns."[7] But as many enthusiasts acknowledged, SCD posed particular clinical and cultural challenges. Most informed observers knew that SCD's therapeutic past had been defined by steady progress. But this history was also replete with sporadic bouts of overpromises, complex therapeutic tradeoffs, and lingering uncertainty among patients and families as to whom or what to believe. Moreover, because of SCD's symbolic significance as a "black disease," researchers had often been quick to seize upon the disease to help draw attention to the sweeping significance of potential breakthroughs for underprivileged African Americans, in much the same way that other researchers might have invoked the whiteness of cystic fibrosis, or pointed to breast cancer among women, in order to give broader social meaning to their own agendas.

By the 1990s, history had taught some sickle cell researchers to be more cautious in their promises of cures and breakthroughs than their peers in the cystic fibrosis research community. In 1993 one popular writer commenting on the future of gene therapy turned his attention to the controversial history of SCD. He cautioned against enthusiasm and against vaunted claims. "Finding a gene and curing a disease are two different things," wrote Bill Deitrich in the *Seattle Times*. For him sickle cell disease was a case in point. Since the late 1940s, scientists had known the cause and had promised therapeutic breakthroughs; Deitrich noted that they "linked sickle-cell disease to a recessive gene in 1948 but are still struggling to find a cure."[8] In the 1990s, sickle cell researchers agreed that breakthroughs aimed at the underlying cause of SCD had been envisioned for decades, and they often urged restraint in light of this history of largely unfulfilled promises. A distinct cultural ethos surrounded SCD, and this ethos would shape public debate about the ups and downs of basic medical care, and about the likelihood of revolutions to come.

THE ARCHETYPAL "MOLECULAR DISEASE"

Like cystic fibrosis, sickle cell disease went from being a relatively obscure disease to a well-known disorder midway through the twentieth century. First conceptualized as a discrete disease in the 1910s and 1920s, SCD had been observed from the very beginning to be especially prevalent among African Americans. The malady was defined by a particular set of symptoms: intense joint pain, lethargy, deadly infections, leg ulcers, and, all too frequently, early childhood death from infectious disease, pneumonia, and the like.[9] After its discovery by Chicago physician James Herrick in 1910, SCD was widely portrayed as a rare disorder. Doctors rarely recognized the death of a sickle cell patient for what it was, for they commonly perceived the symptoms or complications of the disease to be the cause of death. As with cystic fibrosis, in which infections caused the mortality, it would be several decades before physicians cultivated the tools and the habits of mind to distinguish between general cases of pneumonia or of infectious disease and the specific underlying pathologies of CF or SCD. For this reason, in the 1930s and 1940s an obscure malady like sickle cell remained significant only for specialists who took an interest in rare hematological (blood) disorders. SCD attracted little attention among most American physicians, and when these doctors did take notice, there was little discussion of therapy. Linus Pauling's work radically altered this dynamic, introducing the possibility of molecular-level diagnosis and transforming an obscure malady into an "archetypal disease."

The 1949 discovery by Pauling and his colleagues that hemoglobin—the large oxygen-carrying molecules inside red blood cells—played a major role in the formation of sickled red blood cells pointed not only to the mechanism of sickle cell disease but also to the possibility of a cure.[10] As in the history of cystic fibrosis, these new insights into the underlying pathology of SCD gave rise rather quickly to grandiose prospects for a revolutionary therapy. Pauling's work on the abnormal hemoglobin molecule in sickled blood cells gave rise to an intense faith in the possibility of a technical fix for SCD, just as the discovery and cloning of a gene would do for CF years later. An ideology of cure emerged around SCD in the 1950s, built around Pauling's characterization of this malady as a molecular disease. In effect, the idea that SCD was reducible to abnormal hemoglobin made it possible to imagine crafting an enzyme to desickle the crumpled hemoglobin molecule, allowing it to do its job of carrying oxygen from lungs to tissue.

In the wake of the 1949 discovery, it seemed only logical (and not at all fantastic) to envision a new era in molecular medicine, a reductionist medicine focused on curing the disease by creating an enzyme and fixing the hemoglobin. The only question that remained was how this vision would be carried out. Which enzyme would work? What mechanism would be used to alter the molecule? This simple reductionist philosophy—the idea that discrete molecular-level anomalies caused disease—was, at the time, revolutionary. It spurred the growth of a new field of molecular biology, and within a few years the discovery of the structure of DNA by Watson and Crick would draw even more attention to how "primary" molecular-level interactions explained disease processes.

In the case of sickle cell disease, which soon became known as the first "molecular disease," the implications of this reductionist philosophy would play out over decades of laboratory experiments and clinical experiments. In contrast, the reductionist hopes surrounding gene therapy in cystic fibrosis would play out over a far shorter time span—less than a decade—and would come much later. Thus, by the 1990s, when these reductionist hopes were profoundly new for CF patients and their doctors, SCD patients, doctors, and families had already gone through their own vogue for such cures, experiencing bouts of optimism and extraordinary disappointment over the often-repeated promise of an innovative, imminent cure.

As with cystic fibrosis, the antibacterial revolution of the late 1940s and 1950s also had a dramatic impact on the health of sickle cell patients and on the visibility of the disease. In the late 1940s the electrophoretic analysis of hemoglobin molecules pioneered by Pauling and his colleagues opened up the real possibility of a molecular diagnosis for this malady. Simultaneously, antibiotics provided effective treatments for the infections responsible for most of the early childhood mortality. By the 1950s, therefore, SCD had attained a higher profile that paralleled the increasing visibility of cystic fibrosis; indeed, both were "new" children's diseases. Like CF, SCD was transformed from a rare disease of limited interest in the research community into a much more prevalent and scientifically interesting disorder.[11]

In the years before Pauling and penicillin, physicians had experimented with a variety of treatments with little success, including transfusion, removal of the spleen, and various drug regimens; but the events of the 1940s and 1950s set in motion a search for new kinds of treatments—so-called desickling agents—that promised to revolutionize sickle cell care and eradicate suffering and death among African-American children. As one scientist forecast in 1951, "[We] may be able to devise a small innocuous molecule which will lock permanently on to the defective hemoglobin and prevent the abnormal molecule from misbehaving."[12]

Such scientists, like the "gene doctors" two generations later, ardently believed that technical ingenuity would soon result in a complete victory over hereditary disease. The search for such agents was fully engaged by the mid-1950s, but it gained momentum during the 1960s, when Civil Rights struggles and social unrest helped define the "pain and suffering" of SCD as a microcosm of the African-American condition.[13] As this reductionist agenda grew in both scientific and cultural importance, the search for desickling agents attained a particularly high profile in the early 1970s. Pressure grew for national legislation addressing the SCD problem, and Congress and the Nixon administration rallied behind passage of the 1972 National Sickle Cell Anemia Control Act. In this context, urea came to prominence as the long-sought desickling agent. The search for such an agent attracted much attention, but for SCD researchers and patients it quickly revealed the limits of naïve reductionism and the hidden dangers of innovative yet unproven therapies.

THE UREA DEBACLE: THE LIMITS OF REDUCTIONISM IN THE 1970S

The early 1970s marked the peak of national attention to sickle cell disease, a once-obscure disorder that had risen to prominence as a painful "discriminating disease" in which "99% of . . . U.S. victims are black." At the same time, a promising treatment appeared on the horizon. This novel therapy, urea, promised to be the molecular "cure" that the molecular disease demanded. Urea's promoters saw it not only as relief for the patient but also as the fulfillment of the long search. By 1974, however, urea had followed a path akin to the one adenovirus gene therapy would later follow. SCD researchers discovered toxic side effects and widely rejected urea on those grounds, and for years to come the urea episode would remain etched in their memories.

Urea appeared to answer the pressing needs of the moment—a breakthrough medicine for African-American suffering. Late in

1970 a Michigan researcher named Robert Nalbandian announced that he had given doses of urea to two sickle cell patients and that the drug had resulted in the restoration of the sickled cells to normal shape. "The approach," noted another researcher at the time, was "chemically rational and very promising."[14] Quickly, the national media seized upon these developments, suggesting that the discovery "offered new relief for sickle-cell sufferers." Reports described the drug as if it were ready for widespread everyday use. "By treating the patient with a solution of urea and invert sugar," *Time* magazine reported, ". . . the sickling tendency can be reversed and the misshapen cells returned to normal."[15] But researchers knew that urea was a substance that carried severe risks. Nalbandian, for example, cautioned about the danger of dehydration and warned that other effects of the drug had yet to be documented. Many other researchers were quick to point out that Nalbandian's study was not a clinical trial but merely a report on a few "in-house" cases.

The urea findings, and Nalbandian's claims about a therapeutic breakthrough, immediately stirred controversy. Hematologists greeted the announcement of this treatment with a "frosty assessment."[16] As the *Medical World News* reported in January 1971, researchers were split between those who applauded Nalbandian's logical and daring initiative and those who regretted the premature celebration of an unproven drug. At one professional meeting, "charges of irresponsibility and sensationalism met with countercharges of scientific ignorance and illiteracy." For some researchers, the publicity itself was a big part of the problem. One critic commented that "as a result of the widespread publicity, I am afraid that some people are trying this therapy without proper guidance." Others were more strident in their criticism, labeling Nalbandian's press conference on urea "terribly premature" and even "disgraceful." Urea's defenders noted that Nalbandian's news briefing had been misunderstood and that he had called it "primarily to find support for further urea trials," not to promote urea as a therapeutic breakthrough.[17]

The significance of this controversy was clear to a number of reporters, who saw that it typified molecular biology's avid pursuit of a "chemically rational and very promising" therapy while also highlighting the cautiousness of a research culture skeptical of inflated, premature claims. By mid-1971, reporters were describing the use of urea as highly controversial. As for Nalbandian and his team, they were described as having scaled back their claims of breakthrough, now saying that their research was "controversial and too preliminary to talk about in terms of possible treatment of the disease in the human body." There were simply too many unresolved issues. Foremost among them was "toxicity," which remained "an unanswered question." [18]

Over the next few months scientists and the media subjected Nalbandian's "breakthrough" to ever closer scrutiny and criticism. In late 1971 a follow-up study reported on the problems of urea and the severe challenge of even carrying out a proper evaluation of the earlier findings. "Properly controlled studies using the double-blind technique are difficult" the study reported, "because the diuresis [increased secretion of urine] produced by urea may unblind both the patient and the observer after two or three hours and 120 to 150 g of urea." In other words, urea's severe diuretic effects made it obvious to researchers and subjects alike whether the drug or the placebo had been administered, and this knowledge tainted the study by potentially influencing their behavior, biasing their conclusions, and destabilizing any conclusions about the drug's actual worth. By late 1971 it had become clear that diuresis was not merely a nagging methodological complication in the research effort; it was also "a major and potentially dangerous side effect," and there was already evidence that "the death of a child with sickle-cell disease may have been partly related to the dehydration resulting from a massive diuresis for which there was inadequate therapeutic compensation." [19]

By mid-1972, observations about urea's extreme side effects had cast doubt on the drug's clinical efficacy and safety; other laboratory studies had even cast doubt on its capacity to desickle cells, regardless of the side effects.[20] Then in early 1973, uncontrolled clinical trials of urea on eleven patients announced definitively that "no hematologic or clinical benefit could be observed."[21] The era of urea's celebrated promise was ending. By 1974, some of those who in 1970 had expressed admiration for the chemical rationality of the urea "cure" now admitted that it was a failure. A multi-institution study published in the *Journal of the American Medical Association* in May 1974 was the final word, finding "that urea was ineffective in relieving the acute pain that afflicts those suffering from this incurable, hereditary blood disease." The study had also considered a number of other promising agents, comparing them with a placebo, and concluded that "neither urea, nor alkali administration was found to be superior to invert sugar alone in shortening the crisis episode."[22]

Urea enjoyed a brief celebrity in the glaring spotlight of 1970s SCD politics, and its appeal at the time is easy to explain. On one hand, urea fulfilled the longstanding need for "a small, innocuous molecule which will lock permanently on to the defective hemoglobin and prevent the abnormal molecule from misbehaving."[23] On the other hand, insofar as SCD was a microcosm of African-American pain and suffering, urea symbolized relief at last for an ongoing crisis in American race relations and health care. As President Richard Nixon proclaimed when promoting sickle cell disease legislation in 1971, "It is a sad and shameful fact that the causes of this disease have been largely neglected throughout our history. We cannot rewrite this record of neglect, but we can reverse it."[24] Urea's failure, then, represented a disappointment on several levels. After the urea bubble collapsed, few experts on SCD would be so naïve as to accept unquestioningly the idea of a surgically precise molecular cure. Though appealing in the abstract, this sort of idea for rational therapeutics proved difficult to translate into safe and truly effective drugs.

The failure of urea in the early 1970s was a well-publicized blow to an entire research agenda. Indeed, urea was only the most public failure in the effort to create desickling agents; many other agents were promoted, studied, and prematurely celebrated for their desickling qualities.[25] In 1974, for example, a report on the much touted sodium cyanate noted that "the evaluation of the overall clinical efficacy of cyanate is extremely difficult because of the nature of sickle-cell disease." In other words, the complexity of SCD made it difficult to evaluate the benefits of any single agent. As the researchers pointed out, "The three major expressions of the hemoglobinopathy [of SCD] are hemolytic anemia, organ damage, and episodes of pain called 'crises.'" According to their assessment, cyanate performed well in only one of these areas, showing positive effects only on hemolytic anemia.[26] Sodium cyanate failed on the other two fronts, and other researchers concluded that "at the present time cyanate therapy for sickle-cell anemia can only be described as a hopeful new approach awaiting further evaluation to determine its clinical usefulness."[27] Certainly this was not the molecular cure that SCD patients and doctors had been expecting.

Despite the disappointing results with urea and sodium cyanate, the pursuit of rational and chemically appealing drugs did not end—and neither did the controversy. Even after the apparently conclusive 1974 trials on urea, Nalbandian continued to defend his earlier results. He attacked "flaws" in the 1974 trials and insisted that the truth of his original claims "has never been challenged and still holds." He insisted that other researchers had failed to follow his study's protocols to the letter: "Where our protocols have been faithfully followed, there has not been a therapeutic failure, a medical misadventure, or a death."[28] His critics responded that although the protocols were not followed, the fundamental issue was to test Nalbandian's hypothesis that "rapid elevation of the blood urea concentration . . . would abort a sickle cell crisis." This hypothesis was found, without question, to be groundless. "The urea hypothesis," they concluded, "has been tested and found wanting."[29] For the time being, a cure or even relief of the painful "crises" of SCD would have to depend on something other than urea or any other desickling agent. Many physicians believed that comprehensive management of all the symptoms afflicting the SCD patient was the key to better health. The impact of the urea story would linger into the early 1980s. Many clinical researchers, hematologists, and caregivers emerged from the years-long controversy aware of the limitations of naïve reductionism, wary of news reports, and attuned to the need for well-organized clinical trials to test claims about breakthrough drugs or treatments for sickle cell disease.

The spotlight on this "black disease" added another layer of political meaning to public claims and counterclaims about break-through drugs. In the early-1970s, activists, celebrities, commu-nity leaders, the U.S. Congress, and ultimately President Nixon himself had turned their attention to legislation to address this disorder. For many Americans this attention was logical and jus-tified, since "sickle cell anemia [had] for many years . . . been the victim of neglect."[30] Others viewed the new focus on SCD as a mere concession to racial politics. Some observers in black com-munities regarded the increased attention cynically as well, as a ploy by (predominantly white) scientists, physicians, and politi-cians to garner increased federal support by capitalizing on the social plight of African Americans.[31] As one editorialist noted frankly in 1971, "It can be taken as an axiom of American life, that whenever a good cause comes along, those who would exploit it for their own advantage are never far behind. A case in point is sickle cell anemia."[32] Such cynics were quick to see promises of cure merely as exploitation going by another name.

The actions and words of the experts themselves offered plenty of fuel for cynics. Linus Pauling himself, so closely associated with the discovery of the sickle cell hemoglobin and with the search for a desickling agent, helped stir controversy in 1968 when he wrote, "There should be tattooed on the forehead of every young person a symbol showing possession of the sickle-cell gene or whatever other similar gene . . . that he has been found to possess in a single allele." It seemed clear to many such experts that even as they hoped for cures, identifying would-be parents who both carried the sickle cell trait and counseling them about their 25 percent chance of having a child with SCD would be crucial to controlling the disease in the future. Pauling took the idea to an absurd new level, suggesting that the tattoo would allow people carrying the trait to identify one another early in life. "If this were done," he suggested, "two young people carrying the same seriously defective gene in a single dose would recognize this situation at first sight, and would refrain from falling in love with one another."[33] In the context of the racial politics of the late 1960s and early 1970s, such a suggestion was inflammatory. This outrageous idea nurtured cynicism about genetic screening, suggesting—both at the time and for years to come—that the proponents of genetic counseling and screening were focused more on the control of reproduction and on their own agendas than on promoting health per se in black communities. Pauling's notion and Nalbandian's zealous claims would be remembered, along with other insults. In light of such a history, SCD researchers began approaching innovative treatments with a great deal of caution.[34]

Although in 1970 some experts may have continued to regard sickle cell disease as a simple technical problem that might yield to a technical fix, by mid-decade many had become cautious and acutely aware of the complex clinical and sociological problem that was SCD.[35] To be sure, scientists continued to look for safe, rational desickling methods—experimenting with kidney machines, radio frequency waves, and chemotherapies—in hopes of succeeding where urea had failed.[36] But the failure of urea had produced one tangible benefit: the raising of standards and cultural sensibilities among SCD researchers. First of all, it had become clear that even in desickling, prevention worked better than cure. As one reviewer put it, any antisickling therapy "must almost certainly be prophylactic rather than curative: It is substantially more difficult to depolymerize HbS [the abnormal hemoglobin molecule] than it is to prevent it from depolymerizing in the first place." In addition, the diuretic effects of urea had highlighted the fact that any potential new antisickling agent must be very safe, "since it will be used on a daily basis throughout the patient's life."[37] After urea, safety became a key concern. Therapeutic goals also broadened in the late 1970s and early 1980s beyond a search for cures. As two researchers argued in 1982, the allure of innovative cures had diminished greatly, and "even if a new cure bursts forth," most observers understood that "it would not be as safe and effective as chloroquine for malaria or penicillin for pneumonia." Instead, the researchers concluded that while we wait for cures to come along, "we should try to improve our present means for delivering care."[38]

By the early 1980s, then, at the dawn of the discovery of genes causing cystic fibrosis and other diseases, and amid a groundswell of optimism for gene therapy, the sickle cell research community was just recovering from the disastrous infatuation with urea and desickling agents. The controversies over coercive genetic counseling also resounded in public and professional memory. Any breakthroughs in the management of genetic disease that might emerge in the 1980s and 1990s would be assessed against a backdrop of concern about safety, caution about the dangers of inflated therapeutic promises, and anxiety over the highly charged language attached to this "black disease."

THERAPY AS SOCIAL JUSTICE: PAIN AND INFECTION
CARE IN A "HIGHLY CHARGED ATMOSPHERE"

Even though researchers defined sickle cell disease as a "blood disease" (a hemoglobinopathy), its most disturbing features, from doctors' and patients' perspectives, were the intense recurrent pain and life-threatening infections. During the 1980s, these two realities of SCD—pain and infection—came to dominate clinical and public understanding and to overshadow grand hopes of a cure. The clinical management of pain and infection was never far removed from troubling social issues; in the context of American race politics, debates about the use of narcotics in alleviating pain or expensive antibiotics in combating infections often became ve-

Sickle Cell Disease

"THE ARCHETYPAL MOLECULAR DISEASE"

Understanding of SCD has evolved rapidly since Linus Pauling first characterized it as a molecular disease. Its current scientific and medical profile includes the following characterizations.

Carrier Frequency	1 in 12 African Americans
Disease Incidence	1 in 500 African Americans
Inheritance	Autosomal recessive
Cause	Unlike other autosomal recessive diseases, SCD is less frequently described as a "genetic" disorder than as a "molecular defect." Yet the cause of SCD has been identified as a mutation of the hemoglobin B (HbB) gene on chromosome 11.
Mechanism	Hemoglobin molecules allow red blood cells to carry oxygen through the bloodstream and give those cells their characteristic color. SCD patients have abnormal hemoglobins (hemoglobin S) that stick to one another and form long rodlike structures that cause red blood cells to become rigid and assume a sickle shape. These sickle cells pile up and block the flow of blood through vessels, causing pain and resulting in damage to vital tissue and organs (especially the spleen, kidneys, and liver).
Symptoms	Episodes of acute pain known as "crises" (may include pain in joints, bones, or abdomen), anemia, fever, fatigue, breathlessness, rapid heart rate, susceptibility to infections, delayed growth and puberty, leg ulcers, jaundice, and priapism. Patients have an extremely

	high risk of stroke and can suffer long-term complications such as lung tissue damage and cardiovascular disease.
Diagnosis	Blood tests are available for both the sickle cell trait and the disease. Tests include the standard CBC (complete blood count), the sickle cell test, which can detect the presence or absence of abnormal hemoglobin (HbS), and hemoglobin electrophoresis, which can measure the different types of hemoglobin in the blood.
Treatments	A combination of fluids, painkillers, antibiotics, and blood transfusions are used to treat symptoms and complications of SCD. The antitumor drug hydroxyurea has been shown to be effective in preventing painful crises. Though risky, bone marrow transplantation is an option for some patients that may lead to cure.
Prevention	Prenatal testing for fetuses is possible using amniocentesis or chorionic villi sampling to identify the HbB gene. Carrier testing is available for adults.

hicles for expressing anxiety about "inner city" drug addiction, the rising cost of medical care for the poor, and the pursuit of a health care system that was socially fair and just to African Americans.

The management of infection, in the lungs and other organs, commanded a great deal of attention in sickle cell research in the 1970s and 1980s; it was a crucial issue in basic care. Like their counterparts in cystic fibrosis, SCD doctors began to take a closer look at the extensive use of a wide range of antibiotics to fight the blood infections (septicemia) so common among SCD patients.

Sickle Cell Disease

CONTROVERSIES IN PREVENTION AND THERAPY

At many junctures in the history of SCD, discussions of therapeutics and prevention have been shadowed by controversy. From Linus Pauling's controversial comments in the 1960s on methods to prevent SCD carriers from marrying to debates in the 1990s over bone marrow transplantation and other high-risk interventions, physicians and researchers have vigorously debated the pros and cons. The debate has often intertwined with broader discussions about race, equality, and fairness in American society.

"There should be tattooed on the forehead of every young person a symbol showing possession of the sickle-cell gene or whatever other similar gene . . . that he has been found to possess in a single allele . . . If this were done, two young people carrying the same seriously defective gene in a single dose would recognize this situation at first sight, and would refrain from falling in love with one another."
—Linus Pauling, molecular biology pioneer and
  Nobel Prize laureate, 1968

"It is clear to me that the level of mortality, for a procedure intended to cure a disease that manifests such diverse patient-to-patient phenotypic expression, is clearly unacceptable if marrow transplantation is intended as an across-the-board recommendation . . . [It] is not the physician but the patient who should be making the final decision . . . unfortunately, because the patient usually tends to be very young, this decision will fall on the parent or guardian . . . Is there not room for [parents] taking risk for the wrong reasons? What if some parents or guardians decide on marrow transplantation because they believe they cannot provide appropriate support to their child for socioeconomic reasons?"
—Ronald Nagel, SCD researcher and physician, 1991

"Little would be gained by sickle cell disease patients if they merely traded the morbidity associated with their primary disorder for a new set of disabling symptoms resulting from their treatment."
—Ernest Beutler, hematologist, 1991

> "We heard an argument that a 10% mortality with transplantation may not be acceptable . . . On the other hand, we have heard that the quality of the life for sickle cell patients in many instances is perhaps worse than death . . . This is going to be a very subjective decision . . . Some physicians would demand that marrow grafting have almost a zero risk before it should be undertaken in sickle cell disease. It think that is an excessive requirement."
>
> —E. Donnall Thomas, bone marrow transplantation pioneer and Nobel Prize laureate, 1991

Their discussions focused on the wisdom of using penicillin as a prevention against pneunonoccocal infections. The issue attracted public attention in 1986 when researchers announced that the repeated use of "inexpensive penicillin pills" during infancy helped "those suffering from the disease to get past the first few years of life when they are highly susceptible to the strep infection [septicemia]." These findings emerged so unexpectedly and the "results were so dramatic that researchers stopped the study eight months earlier than planned." In a field in which researchers had grown cautious about inflated promises, some offered muted expressions of hope regarding prophylactic penicillin.[39] As researcher Clarice Reid noted in an interview with *Black Enterprise*, "I don't like to use the word breakthrough . . . But we can now show that this drug therapy (oral penicillin for SCD infants) can make a difference."[40]

Prophylactic penicillin became standard for children with sickle cell disease in the 1980s, but doubts about the practice lingered—among them, questions about the cost. In 1991, for example, Miami-based researchers pointed out that this method was not perfect and that "pneumococcal bacteremia with its resultant high mortality rate must be expected to occur despite the prescription of penicillin prophylaxis."[41] Penicillin did not solve the problem of infections among SCD patients, and the increasing use of antibacterial agents carried significant risks (witness the increasing prevalence of *Pseudomonas* infections among cystic fibrosis patients). Two Dallas-based researchers noted that a regime of prophylactic penicillin was perhaps warranted only for the highest-risk SCD patients: "Young children with SC disease . . . may not require penicillin prophylaxis because . . . they are not at high risk of having pneumococcal septicemia."[42] They insisted that antibiotics should not be a standard part of SCD care but should be evaluated on a case-by-case basis. And as the 1990s ushered in a new era of medical cost-cutting and managed care, the problem with prophylactic penicillin was increasingly regarded as one of expense.

The long-term financial implications of extended antibiotic use, coupled with its variable efficacy and the growing problem of antibiotic-resistant bacteria, conspired against standardized use of prophylactic antibiotics in SCD care. The problem, of course, would have been familiar to CF physicians, for they too were grappling with whether standardized care was even possible, let alone desirable, given the enormous variation from patient to patient and the rise of antibiotic-resistant strains of bacteria. For an increasing number of physicians, hopes for standardized antibacterial care seemed doomed by the resilience of nature itself. As one SCD researcher put it, standardized use of penicillin in "very young children may . . . hasten the emergence of penicillin-resistant strains of S. *pneumoniae* while providing little benefit."[43] Other studies echoed these anxieties, pointing to the "increasing problem of antibiotic-resistant pneumococcal infection in children with sickle cell disease in the U.S."[44]

By late 1995, however, some SCD physicians were insisting that the real issue was not penicillin per se but building a comprehensive system that provided better access to the range of therapies needed for the complex malady. As one observer noted, "Children with sickle cell anemia who are receiving comprehensive care have a low risk of having pneumococcal bacteremia or meningitis regardless of whether or not they continue to receive prophylactic penicillin." Indeed, prophylactic penicillin might even be scaled back where patients had access to a robust system of medical care: "Children with sickle cell anemia who have not had a prior severe pneumococcal infection . . . and are receiving comprehensive care, may safely stop prophylactic penicillin therapy at 5 years of age." [45] Such comments raised the question of whether the particular drugs were the issue or whether the health care system in general was failing poor children.

Because a significant percentage of sickle cell patients were both poor and black, and because programs like Medicaid often financed medical services for this portion of the patient community, questions about the quality of SCD treatment often elided with conservative anxieties about the cost of "welfare" programs and with liberal concerns about achieving racial equality. From one standpoint, the key concern with SCD was containing health care costs and reducing the heavy expense of federal medical programs. From another perspective, the issue was poor people's lack of access to sound health insurance and their difficulties gaining access to care. In 1993, for example, two researchers writing on pain management in hematology insisted that one of the problems of the specialty was that "Medicaid patients . . . received the most expensive class of pain medications at a significantly higher rate than other patients." [46] As for antibiotics, some physicians insisted that the development of outpatient antibacterial therapy for febrile patients with sickle cell disease was a good investment and would bring "substantial reductions in cost." [47] Such discussions of the economics of SCD treatment should be understood as part of the evolving social debates of the 1980s and 1990s over the control of rising costs, the scaling back of federal government programs, and access to health care—all of these being issues with strong racial undercurrents.

As it had in the 1970s, the recurrent and fierce joint, abdominal, and back pain associated with sickle cell disease continued to embody personal and racial meanings in the 1980s and 1990s.

The "painful crises"—pain and suffering long ignored in black America—were perhaps the most important aspect of patients' experience of the disorder, even though pain itself was not a primary cause of mortality. Pain increasingly occupied SCD doctors and patients, in the same way that lung damage had become the primary concern of CF doctors and patients in the 1970s. In both cases patient advocates drew attention, quite naturally, to those features of the disease that they deemed to be most vital. Thus, from the 1970s through the 1990s, pain management in SCD continued to be a top priority for clinical practice and research.

But pain management in sickle cell disease proved to be a difficult and endlessly controversial matter. A central problem was the enduring fear among practitioners of "creating addicts" through the irregular use of narcotic painkillers and analgesics. For many, erring on the side of caution—prescribing fewer narcotics—was the best policy. For others, liberal prescribing was best, for it addressed patients' profound agony and was an index of medicine's compassion. As two thoughtful practitioners noted in the early 1980s, the therapeutic questions overlapped with questions of race relations and cross-cultural understanding: "Sickle cell anemia . . . occurs in black patients who still face obstacles that whites don't appreciate . . . Treatable complaints must be recognized, painful episodes must be managed."[48]

Increasing skepticism about liberal pain management emerged in the 1980s and 1990s, contrasting sharply with attitudes of the 1960s and 1970s, when attention to the social condition of African Americans had first brought the pain of sickle cell disease to public and medical prominence. "Go to any hospital frequented by blacks," noted one author in the 1970s, "and you will see them . . . The one thing they will all have in common is the memory of excruciating pain. Those who are in the hospital are there usually because they have undergone a recent 'crisis.'"[49] Because of such portraits, acute, recurring bouts of pain remained central to the cultural meaning of SCD. Indeed, researchers often measured the efficacy of the new desickling agents by their potential to reduce or eliminate these painful events. Patients often knew better than their doctors what mixture of painkillers worked best for them, and some often required escalating doses to endure the crises. But skepticism about the authenticity of pain also began to creep into clinical discussions. Medicine's inability to measure pain objectively made it necessary for emergency room doctors, nurses, and sickle cell specialists to rely on their own judgment when making decisions about how or whether to treat a patient's pain.[50]

Not surprisingly, in the increasingly conservative 1980s and 1990s, with public skepticism running high about welfare cheats and drug addicts, alternatives to the use of narcotics in pain management occupied the attention of some leading researchers.[51] Pain management in sickle cell disease had always required a broad point of view. As Boston physician Orah Platt noted, a variety of factors now played into how doctors were choosing to treat (or not to treat) sickle cell pain: "The variability and unpredictability of the healing process, the repetitive nature of the pain, the lack of objective signs, the disquieting need for escalating does of narcotic agents, and the well-founded fear of iatrogenic (i.e., medically induced) respiratory suppression, and the less well-founded fear of narcotic addiction contribute to the highly charged atmosphere that often characterizes the care of desperately uncomfortable patients with sickle cell crises."[52] Increasingly, such fears played a leading role in therapeutic choices.

A nurse's skepticism about a patient's pain or a doctor's "fear of narcotic addiction" created formidable obstacles for patients seeking pain relief. Other perceptions also came into play. As one physician noted in 1993, "In this emergency room, because of both the nature of the disease and the nature of the neighborhood we're in (an urban, largely black community), [sickle cell disease is] seen most often in young, poor blacks—the very same population in which we most worry about narcotic addiction in the first place." As such physicians knew, the medical and social anxiety about addiction placed a huge burden on SCD patients: "Add all this up and it becomes way too easy for jaded doctors and nurses to dismiss a young sickle-cell patient as a faker just out to get drugs."[53] Another doctor put it this way: "Before you can get past the agony, you have to convince a doctor that it's real."[54]

As in the story of Tay-Sachs and cystic fibrosis, a particular cultural ethos surrounded sickle cell patient care and gave meaning to the disease. As in CF, therapeutic progress in SCD brought many frustrations. Progress was further complicated by a charged political climate that at every turn changed therapeutic discussions into racial debates. Issues of care became inseparable from broader issues of fairness, compassion, social justice, and racial injustice. But also as in the CF story, there was hope of imminent breakthroughs, and two promising innovations emerged in the late 1980s and the 1990s: a drug (hydroxyurea) promoted as a genetic switch to turn on healthy hemoglobin; and a technique (bone marrow transplantation) to produce healthy blood cells. The appeal of these innovations lay in part in the fact that they both promised technical solutions to the full range of social, cultural, and medical complexities of SCD: if they worked, these methods would make the exceedingly complex social controversies simply go away. Yet even here, previous disappointments with "breakthroughs" brought out the cautiousness now ingrained among SCD professionals and tempered their enthusiasm. Many physicians continued to stress the practical matters—pain management and prophylactic penicillin—that were most crucial in the lives of African Americans with SCD. But some doctors and researchers still hoped for a true breakthrough. As a profile of researcher Clarice Reid noted in 1988, "Although oral penicillin serves as an effective treatment, [she] sees two other possibilities: bone marrow transplantation and gene therapy."[55] Alongside frustrations with the political complexities of SCD care, there also ran hope that such new developments might sweep away these contentious issues once and for all.

Hydroxyurea (HU), a drug used for treating leukemia, brought genetic medicine to the bedside of sickle cell patients in the 1990s, and its immediate appeal as a treatment for SCD stemmed in no small part from its purported ability to address many of the socio-medical issues that complicated patients' lives. Hydroxyurea was something new, it was said. It was part of a new class of drugs that apparently held out the same "dazzling promise" as had urea and the other therapeutic breakthroughs of the 1970s, but without the side effects. In the early 1990s, HU was greeted by the popular media and professionals alike as part of the revolution in genetic medicine, for it was said to work like a "genetic switch" for regulating the production of nonsickling red blood cells. Adding to its appeal, the drug also showed promise for reducing the number of painful episodes that patients suffered, thereby diminishing the need for hospitalization and saving patients, insurers, and the health care system money in the long run. When HU appeared in the 1990s, it thus seemed to be an ideal drug for addressing SCD at every level—at the molecular and genetic level, at the level of the patient's experience, in the clinic, and also in the larger economy of SCD care.

The advent of HU reflected two developments in genetic medicine. The first was the growing use of recombinant DNA techniques in drug production. The second was the emergence of what would become known as genetic drug therapies: a class of drugs that apparently turned genes on, turned them off, regulated their production of proteins, or (in the case of gene therapy) altered them by replacing parts of the DNA. The first of these promising genetic drugs therapies for sickle cell disease—a kind of precursor to HU—had appeared in the early 1980s. In December 1982 a *Newsweek* article entitled "Switch on Genes" hailed the recent findings on 5-azacytidine. Basing its report on a study published in the *New England Journal of Medicine*, *Newsweek* noted that researchers had given this well-known cancer drug to patients with SCD and beta-thalassemia and had witnessed "a sharp rise in hemoglobin levels and . . . improvement in symptoms."[56] *Time* magazine reported that 5-azacytidine worked by reactivating "apparently intact genes that had been dormant since birth" so as to produce fetal hemoglobin cells. This was a crucial development, since fetal hemoglobin cells did not sickle as did adult hemoglobin. The drug apparently worked like a switch to activate the production of cells that had last been seen in the patient's infancy.

In keeping with the rising expectations of the time, the *Time* article looked forward to the day when "genetic switches" would be followed by new forms of "genetic surgery," a future in which doctors would eventually "use recombinant DNA techniques to cut out 'bad' genes and substitute 'good' ones." Echoing the forward-looking, optimistic beliefs of genetic researchers, such popular accounts saw 5-azacytidine as a harbinger of medicine to come, "a major new step in treating disease [that] demonstrates beyond doubt that genetic manipulation has come to the bedside."[57] For the remainder of the 1980s, researchers speculated openly about the "long-term goal of gene therapy for sickle cell disease," a goal that seemed quite attainable, awaiting only "additional technical advances for increasing the efficiency of gene transfer and the level of gene expression."[58] Longtime SCD researchers acknowledged that "replacing defective genes with normal ones [would be] 'the ultimate therapy.'"[59] Yet SCD researchers also knew that 5-azacytidine was not an ideal genetic switch. The safety of the 5-azacytidine compound remained in question throughout the 1980s, and when SCD researchers learned that the agent was carcinogenic in laboratory animals, the enthusiasm for this particular cancer drug quickly disappeared.

The failure of 5-azacytidine to prove itself a viable drug for sickle cell disease did not, however, dampen enthusiasm for less toxic compounds that might act as a genetic switch for producing nonsickling hemoglobin cells. Hydroxyurea, a drug often used in the treatment of leukemia and the blood disorder polycythemia vera, now moved into the spotlight. Like 5-azacytidine, HU had been shown to increase fetal hemoglobin production in SCD patients. The goal of HU therapy was not to cure the disease; in the words of Johns Hopkins researcher Samuel Charache, it was "to produce a milder form of sickle cell disease in adults by increasing the levels of fetal hemoglobin." But it remained unclear whether HU could actually do the job reliably, said Charache. "The treatment works very well for some patients and not at all for others, but we don't know why." In view of these and other uncertainties, six medical centers had begun clinical trials on HU in the late 1980s. The studies sought to examine the impact of HU not only on fetal hemoglobin production but also on the frequency of painful episodes. Within months, the trials had begun to confirm what researchers like Charache suspected: HU worked. Yet, as he noted cautiously, "we have never precisely defined what crises are and placebo effects are very powerful, so even though it came out the way we'd like, this doesn't really mean anything. We have to do a controlled trial before anyone is going to believe that HU does anything for these patients." He also warned that HU was still considered a "dangerous drug."[60]

Such words of caution could not stand in the way of popular and professional endorsement of HU as another promising "genetic switch." Even though HU's value lay in its potential to reduce the number of crises or, as Charache had said, to produce a "milder form of SCD," some saw this "genetic switch" as a revolutionary break from all other therapies.[61] "For the first time," stated NIH researcher Griffin Rodgers, "we're treating the underlying disease, instead of simply the complications." The "genetic" label became affixed to HU, placing it in a separate category of therapy from existing treatments for pain and infection. HU promised to accomplish what urea and the other desickling agents had been unable to do. Rodgers and others insisted, however, that their enthusiasm should not be interpreted as premature endorsement, since these results were still preliminary: "At the current time, treatment with such agents such as HU and/or recombinant human erythropoetin should be considered experimental, and efforts should be made to enroll eligible patients into ongoing clinical trials, where possible." [62] Other researchers cautioned that "several issues of hydroxyurea therapy remain unresolved, including differences in patients' drug clearance, predictability of drug response, reversibility of sickle cell disease–related organ damage by hydroxyurea, and the efficacy of elevated HbF [fetal hemoglobin]." [63] In 1994 even Charache noted that there were many anomalies about HU—among them, the odd fact that "crises decreased during treatment, but this decrease was noted before the HbF levels increased." [64] The growing optimism for this new "genetic switch" was thus counterbalanced by questions about the actual value of HU for the total experience of SCD: pain, infection, early mortality, strokes, and so on. Researchers remained circumspect about HU even as they embraced its properties as a "genetic switch."

Dramatic confirmation of HU's value came in early 1995 when Charache announced that the Bristol-Myers drug had been judged highly effective in reducing the number of crises—so effective, in fact, that the multicenter clinical trials had been halted abruptly. Charache remained cautious, however. In a field too often given to hyperbole and inflated rhetoric about "breakthroughs" and "cures," he stressed that "we want to emphasize that hydroxyurea is a treatment for the disease and not a cure." The trials confirmed that HU had "reduced by 50 percent the number of pain episodes [experienced by patients, as well as] hospitalizations, situations requiring blood transfusion and incidents of a life-threatening complication called acute chest syndrome, which is characterized by fever and severe chest pain." There was little question that the drug made life with the disease a bit more bearable; but the disease remained. And the trials also raised questions that would not be answered for years to come. In 1995, for instance, "the only adverse effect [then known] was that high dose hydroxyurea caused the suppression of bone marrow, which makes blood cells [and that this effect] might increase the risk of a type of leukemia." [65]

As with 5-azacytidine, the long-term risk of cancer loomed. Medical use of the breakthrough drug would entail the same kind of risk-benefit calculus that had shaped the long history of SCD care from the rise and fall of urea into the age of 5-azacytidine and prophylactic penicillin.

The HU trials also drew public attention to the significant economic interests of drug companies, researchers, and patients in the new drug. In January 1995 a *Wall Street Journal* article noted that the clinical trials were a crucial milestone for the drug's manufacturer, since "until it is approved, Bristol-Myers is forbidden from marketing the drug for the malady, but yesterday's announcement [of the halting of the trial] is expected—indeed, intended—to encourage doctors treating patients with severe forms of the disease to prescribe it."[66] Charache hoped that following this announcement, the Food and Drug Administration would quickly approve the drug, a move that might, he believed, persuade insurance companies to provide coverage so that physicians would be reimbursed for using HU. "If a third-party payer says he's not going to pay until the drug is approved, it will leave a lot of patients out in the cold," Charache stated. The clinical trials were significant for multiple groups—patients, drug companies, doctors, and insurers—and were instrumental in bringing the new drug to the marketplace and to the bedside. HU was an exemplary instance of "basic research [reaching] the clinic, and many observers waited eagerly for the drug to come into wider use."[67]

In late 1996, as HU was becoming increasingly integrated into the care of sickle cell patients, a familiar pattern emerged: researchers now turned to the problem of long-term adverse consequences, and their optimism gave way to more cautious pronouncements. Writing in the pages of the *Hematology Oncology Clinics of North America*, Charache commented that the "long-term risks are worrisome." Researchers had confirmed that "development of leukemia [in patients with polycythemia vera] was more common in patients treated with hydroxyurea."[68] The status of HU therapy in SCD continued to be debated into the late 1990s and through 2004. Most researchers stood by its positive effects on the crises, but they also worried about the long-term risk of leukemia—dangers that were evident quite early in the history of the "genetic switch" drug.

Hydroxyurea provided yet another example of what had become a recurring theme in the ups and downs of therapy for sickle cell disease. There were, it seemed, no true and lasting breakthroughs without long-term costs; there were no radical, transformative cures, only perilous tradeoffs. As in the story of gene therapy for cystic fibrosis, there were significant financial interests in HU. But whereas CF researchers saw gene therapy as a breakthrough cure and embraced the idea of complete disease transformation, SCD researchers viewed HU (as Charache had noted) through a more cautious lens. At best, HU was a drug that produced "a milder form of SCD." Its users would not find cures; rather, they would be walking a new and perilous therapeutic tightrope if they could get access to the new drugs. For many doctors and patients, a kind of sobriety about curative claims had become part of the ethic of care. Not surprisingly, then, the promise of bone marrow transplantation for SCD would also prompt concerns. What unseen dangers and tradeoffs lay hidden in this innovative venture?

A DANGEROUS WAY OUT: THE BONE MARROW TRANSPLANT LOTTERY

The use of bone marrow transplantation (BMT) to treat sickle cell disease represented an extreme version of the perilous therapeutic situation posed by hydroxyurea—not so much a tightrope as a perverse therapeutic lottery. The lottery metaphor is an apt one. As the bone marrow transplantation option emerged in the early 1990s, it raised intense debate about whether the extraordinary risks of the procedure made it too dangerous to offer patients and families, even if its benefits were also extraordinary. The discussion about BMT for sickle cell disease had curious parallels to the simultaneous public discussion about lotteries in general. As one 1992 editorial in the St. Louis Post-Dispatch put it, "Blacks and Hispanics consistently play lotteries more frequently than whites. Many state lotteries have even devised separate marketing strategies aimed at black and Hispanic players in what can only be described as a despicable attempt to plunder two already economically oppressed minorities."[69] The questions that emerged around BMT, although they were cast in the muted tones of academic discussion, followed similar lines as American debates over state lotteries. Was this high-risk gamble a heroic way out of a life of frustration, poverty, and pain? Or was it a false dream, a tragic form of exploitation?

In late 1984 national media sources reported that "doctors have cured a case of sickle cell anemia with a bone marrow transplant." Such reports fanned out across the broadcast spectrum, but below the headlines they cautioned that "this life-saving therapy will be suitable for only a small minority of victims of the disease" and that "the transplants [are] fatal about 30 percent of the time."[70] An array of limiting factors meant that not all patients with SCD but only a minority of them would be suitable candidates for BMT. The crucial qualifying factor was that transplantation required the availability of donors with matching bone marrow, usually siblings or close relatives. But such matches—human leukocyte antigen (HLA) matches—were not assured even among family members. Even when HLA-matched donors could be arranged, embedded in the technology was a troubling conundrum. BMT offered the possibility of unambiguous "cure" from SCD, but it also came with high risks of death during the procedure. From the outset, then, reports on BMT and sickle cell disease provoked controversy. Even amid the excitement about the single patient who had been cured, researchers' optimism was constrained by the moral and ethical complexity of this risky advance.[71]

There were other troubling problems with using BMT in sickle cell disease. Researchers were aware of one long-term consequence: the likelihood (also high) that patients would be neither cured nor killed but would develop "major immunological complications, particularly graft-vs.-host disease, which currently limit[s] the more widespread use of marrow transplantation in the therapy of sickle cell anemia." Graft-versus-host disease (GVHD), a profound and often devastating immunological attack by the transplanted organ (the graft) on the recipient (the host), could often (though not always) be managed as a chronic disease. This potential outcome amounted to the replacement of one chronic condition (SCD) with another (GVHD). GVHD could also be fatal.

For all of these reasons, bone marrow transplantation remained highly controversial and extraordinarily limited in its appeal. Certainly, its impact on overall rates of sickle cell disease would be slight. Debate on the ethics of offering the procedure to patients and families roiled the hematology field through the 1980s. As two researchers noted in 1989, "The use of this technique at its present stage of development for the treatment of . . . sickle cell anemia . . . is controversial, raises serious ethical issues, and cannot be recommended routinely at this time."[72] The risk-benefit calculus surrounding BMT forced sickle cell patients and their hematologists to weigh the benefit of this potential "cure" against the relatively high probabilities of another costly chronic disease and even death.

The intense debate about the pros and cons of bone marrow transplantation continued into the 1990s.[73] Many hematologists had come together at an August 1990 conference at the Fred Hutchinson Cancer Research Center in Seattle, Washington, to discuss the new "cure" that was causing such a stir in the field. For many, the question of BMT came back to the question of what physicians owed to their patients, what risks and choices ought to be offered to them, and whether BMT should be understood as an "experiment" or as an "innovative therapy." The conference, not surprisingly, revealed sharp divisions and conflicting opinions. There were those who believed that dreams of quick cures simply distracted researchers, patients, families, and the public from the goal of providing the comprehensive care—the management of infections, pain, and symptoms—that truly advanced the lives of most SCD patients but that still eluded far too many. For these researchers, it was more appropriate to think about therapeutic advances that benefited larger numbers rather than troubling breakthroughs for the few. And then there were those who advocated the path of dramatic risk-taking. For them, BMT was a bold step in the long pursuit of significant breakthroughs. Considering that the researchers could not agree among themselves about the appropriateness of BMT, it should come as no surprise that they also disagreed strongly on the question of how this option should be presented (if at all) to SCD patients, research subjects, and their families.

Such explicit professional discussion of the risks and purported benefits of bone marrow transplantation stood in dramatic contrast to the discussions then unfolding in the world of cystic fibrosis. CF was becoming increasingly known as a Caucasian malady. As we saw in the previous chapter, there were exalted expectations among CF patients, physicians, and researchers of an imminent gene therapy breakthrough. Hopes ran high; experimental risks were embraced; and new entrepreneurial ventures promised huge profits for venture capitalists and longer, healthier lives for CF patients. A very different and far less optimistic sensibility surrounded SCD. By now it should be clear that dramatically different historical experiences shaped this sensibility. There were many past controversies to reflect upon, numerous promises made and unfulfilled; there were the fraught meanings of "experimentation" in the black community and lingering questions about the high price and limited impact of innovation for patients; and finally, there was frustration about the widespread lack of access to basic care. The troubling legacy of stigma, the fears of exploitation, and the cynicism of many African Americans about SCD care emerged directly out of therapeutic encounters; ambivalence, wariness, and skepticism grew, quite naturally, alongside every promise of cure.

In their reflections on the bone marrow transplantation question, many sickle cell researchers looked back over the history of promises and setbacks and voiced their by-now ingrained caution. Speaking of the effects of BMT in Cooley's anemia, one researcher noted that "bone marrow transplantation was associated with as much as 25% mortality and the event-free survival was as low as 65%." At the very least, he noted, "one has to be selective of the type of patient that can be transplanted, rather than transplant all patients indiscriminately."[74] Ronald Nagel, a New York–based physician, agreed: "It is clear to me that the level of mortality, for a procedure intended to cure a disease that manifests such diverse patient-to-patient phenotypic expression, is clearly unacceptable if marrow transplantation is intended as an across-the-board recommendation."[75] Not only were mortality risks too high, he suggested, but the variability in how SCD manifested itself in patients made it all the more difficult to determine which patients should be offered this roll of the dice.

These cautious comments revealed that the calculations and tradeoffs inherent in many other therapeutic modalities had become explicit, and impossible to ignore, with the advent of bone marrow transplantation. Researchers still had imprecise knowledge about variations from patient to patient—with respect to pain, anemia, or other clinical problems—and it was unclear how these variations should inform the evaluation of new drugs and procedures. Yet another problem made obvious by the BMT question was that some therapies offering "cures" were in reality only offering patients the possibility of "trading one disease for another." This was not unlike the dilemma confronting cystic fibrosis physicians and patients as they weighed the tradeoffs between fewer infections and the danger of antibacterial-resistant organisms, between fatal lung deterioration and a new life of medical dependence as a lung transplantee. The BMT tradeoff in sickle cell disease seemed particularly stark and tragic. As hematologist Ernest Beutler summed it up, "Little would be gained by sickle cell disease patients if they merely traded the morbidity associated with their primary disorder for a new set of disabling symptoms resulting from their treatment."[76]

Despite the generally cautious appraisal of bone marrow transplantation, one subset of researchers embraced risk-taking and bold forays into BMT experimentation. Among them was E. Donnall Thomas, awarded the Nobel Prize for his use of bone marrow transplantation in treating leukemia, and a man who had faced criticism early in his leukemia research for taking undue risks with seriously ailing children. Not surprisingly, he spoke in favor of risk-taking. "We heard an argument that a 10% mortality with transplantation may not be acceptable," he began. "On the other hand," he continued, "we have heard that the quality of the life for sickle cell patients in many instances is perhaps worse than death." There was no simple answer to the conundrum. "This is going to be a very subjective decision," he conceded, yet the holding back of innovative therapies because they posed a risk was deeply problematic. For Thomas, the goal of zero risk was unrealistic: "Some physicians would demand that marrow grafting have almost a zero risk before it should be undertaken in sickle cell disease. I think that is an excessive requirement."[77]

The debate among experts over bone marrow transplantation in sickle cell disease touched on such issues as what constituted acceptable risk, but there was something deeply disturbing about the broader context in which such choices would be made. Many experts understood that one of the most troubling questions was who would be making these choices. Who would be accepting the terms of this life-and-death lottery? Nagel stated that "it is not the physician but the patient who should be making the final decision." But this was itself a troubled proposition, since "unfortunately, because the patient usually tends to be very young, this decision will fall on the parent or guardian. The role of the physician . . . is to provide the most objective, dispassionate, and informed counseling in which the available data are presented in clear terms, and with the appropriate caveats as to their application to individual cases."[78] Leaving such decisions to parents or guardians would not solve any problems. Nagel wondered about the role socioeconomic circumstances might play in families' decisions. Could desperate poverty influence their therapeutic decisions for the worse? "Is there not room for [parents] taking risk for the wrong reasons? What if some parents or guardians decide on marrow transplantation because they believe they cannot provide appropriate support to their child for socioeconomic reasons?"[79]

Such questions reveal yet again the fundamental connections between sickle cell therapeutics and broader issues of social justice—connections that some SCD researchers had grown adept at making. Indeed, for some observers the crucial question about bone marrow transplantation was not how researchers weighed the probabilities and statistics but rather the ethical and moral problem of presenting this option in the first place to families who were in disadvantaged social circumstances and who often had trouble getting even basic care. The costs of a one-time fix (even if successful) were weighed not only against the likelihood of death and the long-term costs of caring for a child with GVHD, but also against what an equivalent dollar amount would accomplish if put into comprehensive care and improving access to conventional SCD care. Where strong comprehensive care facilities were lacking and where parents were frustrated about the costs of long-term SCD care, could it be considered fair practice to offer the lottery of BMT? Indeed, rather than pushing questions of justice and fairness into the background, BMT rather dramatically accentuated concerns that had always surrounded SCD care.

The BMT option posed a variety of perplexing new ethical dilemmas as well. To what extent should professionals and experts control these decisions, and to what extent should patients decide for themselves? Should such choices be dictated by market forces alone? These were ethical problems, to be sure, each carrying a particular political resonance in the market-oriented, patient-activist context of the 1980s and 1990s. Questions about the purported virtue of the marketplace and the problem of regulation roiled American society throughout the 1980s and 1990s. Beginning with the deregulatory zeal of the Reagan era and continuing into the 1990s under President Clinton, these years witnessed heated debate about the deregulation of scientific research. Did regulation provide vital protection for research subjects, or was it merely so much red tape standing in the way of progress?

For some, the controversy surrounding bone marrow transplantation was an extension of this larger discussion. In the late 1980s and early 1990s, for example, several researchers at the University of Chicago, a major transplantation center, apparently became frustrated by the ethical questions that, they believed, stood in the way of bringing BMT to sickle cell patients and families. Denied approval by their own institutional review board (IRB) to conduct BMT trials for sickle cell disease, they sought an evidence-based solution: they turned to the market of potential consumers —the families of children with SCD—and asked what they wanted and what they thought constituted an acceptable risk. The idea was to hand the decision over to families, to document their concerns, to study which kinds of families might opt for the risks of BMT and which might not, and to use this knowledge to guide the future use of BMT.

The Chicago researchers published their findings in the *New England Journal of Medicine*, offering their study as a portrait of the prospective consumers of bone marrow transplantation: a risk-taking subset of families with SCD children. They found that "at least 13 percent of parents might be expected to consent . . . given current rates of morbidity and mortality," and that these parents did not harbor the same concerns as the university's own cautious IRB members. These risk-taking parents apparently "weighed the risks and benefits of bone marrow transplantation . . . in a different way from members of our institutional review board." Studying the demographic profile of these parents, the researchers found revealing patterns. The families tended to have female children with SCD, and they tended to have attained higher levels of formal education. As the researchers noted, educational level mattered: "Parents who had graduated from high school were significantly more likely to accept some risk in exchange for cure than those who were not high-school graduates." And parents who remained at home with their children were less likely to embrace the risk: "Parents who were employed or in school were more likely to accept some risk than those who were not occupied outside the home." The findings seemed to suggest that BMT did not exploit the desperation of the poor; rather, it appealed to better-off families with more formal education, those who had presumably come to share the values and aspirations of the American middle-class mainstream. Having identified these risk-taking families, the researchers argued that it was only natural for IRBs to remove the ethical obstacles, allowing physicians and surgeons to target specific black families willing to accept the risk of BMT. They did not address the gender question—why families with girls were more inclined to roll the dice on BMT—which for some would itself have raised profound ethical concerns. Nor did they discuss the implications of tilting the practice toward privileged families willing to gamble with their sick children. Despite the researchers' arguments, the question remained: Should medicine be offering these kinds of odds and choices at all? Should such dangerous life-sustaining techniques be part of the American medical marketplace?[80]

Researchers remained divided in the mid-1990s, and the experts held tightly on to the reins of decision making. As two Boston researchers noted in 1996, "Clinicians must now weigh the pros and cons." Bone marrow transplantation offered extraordinary health advantages, they added, for "a successful outcome is definitive, and unless severe, chronic graft-versus-host disease occurs, the procedure is curative." But families also faced the possibility of crushing, permanent loss: "The potential for cure comes at a considerable risk, most of which is incurred at the time of the procedure." Many doctors and researchers found themselves weighing these almost incalculable risks against the relative safety of hydroxyurea therapy. HU was at least adequate for the "humble goal" of reducing crises, and it "could be discontinued" if complications ever appeared.[81] The same could not be said for bone marrow transplantation.

Paralleling in some ways the debate over antibiotics, bone marrow transplantation posed a fiscal dilemma that futher complicated assessments of the procedure. Did the high short-term cost (in dollars as well as lives lost) justify the potential long-term gains for the few able and willing to gamble? As one Newsweek story pointed out, "The transplant costs about $150,000 and is typically covered by insurers [for those with health insurance coverage]." In contrast, "conventional treatment . . . runs roughly $30,000 to $50,000 a year and can only relieve symptoms."[82] This kind of calculation suggested that in sheer monetary terms, the transplant was a wise long-term investment. Charache, among others, acknowledged that "over the lifetime of a . . . patient with moderately severe disease, medical expenses alone are several-fold greater [under conventional care] than the cost of transplant." Indeed, researchers on all sides agreed with Charache that "there is no debate over the cost-efficacy of transplantation if the patient has disease-free survival."[83] Of course, patients with "disease-free survival" constituted (through the 1990s) only a minority of SCD patients on whom BMT was employed. In many ways this was a false calculus for most SCD patients, one that reduced losses and gains to mere money. The more important questions, as many researchers in the SCD community were quick to note, were social: Who would have access to HLA-matched donor marrow? Whose insurance would approve the procedure? And which of this small percentage of SCD patients would survive the dangerous "experimental therapy" to benefit from the economic trade-off?[84] On the first question alone, Charache concluded that "in the United States, only about 18% of [SCD] patients would be expected to have HLA-identical full siblings."[85] In this therapeu-

tic lottery, in other words, not everyone would be able to buy a
ticket.

BETWEEN PROMISE AND PERIL

By the mid-1990s, the conversation about therapeutics and
revolutions in care in sickle cell disease had already endured dramatic ascents and descents along a troubling roller-coaster terrain. Amid the rush of new promises of genetic cures, many hematologists considered the promise as well as the perils of innovative
practice, the ethical conundrums of these therapeutic options,
and (most important) the ways in which these options intersected
with the lives of SCD patients and their families. Even if there was
not full agreement on the ethics of bone marrow transplantation,
the research community had developed an insightful ambivalence
about breakthroughs. What, they asked, did breakthroughs in care
really mean for patients?

Whether the topic was urea or hydroxyurea, pain management
or bone marrow transplantation, discussions about therapy for
sickle cell disease differed markedly in character and tone from
contemporary discussions about cystic fibrosis and Tay-Sachs disease. To be sure, many sickle cell researchers hailed BMT as a
curative breakthrough, yet even here the optimism was decidedly
muted. Ambivalence, skepticism, and caution abounded. Unlike
the CF "gene doctors" who came out of the subculture of research
entrepreneurism, most sickle cell researchers weighing the evidence on BMT had no financial stake in the outcome. On weighing all the evidence, most agreed that BMT remained too risky and
that "the search for other therapies not based on marrow transplantation should be continued."[86] Those who sought to promote
BMT had to sidestep or argue away the ethical problems raised by
the innovative technique. Like those who championed gene therapy in CF, some in the SCD research community endorsed the idea
that innovation should be speedily brought to consumers and that

the regulatory barriers to the use of BMT should be removed.[87] But they were the minority in a culture in which patients, families, and practitioners had grown cautious yet hopeful about easy promises of cure.

At the 1997 meeting of the Sickle Cell Anemia Disease Association, the Boston hematologist-oncologist David Nathan outlined the current state of therapies. He spoke about hydroxyurea for pain management and blood transfusion, and only at the end did his discussion turn to the prospect of "gene therapy." At the same time that other researchers hailed adenoviruses as tailor-made vehicles for delivering genetic material to the lungs of cystic fibrosis patients, no similarly simple experimental delivery system had emerged for SCD gene therapy. A decade earlier, researchers had promised that "the long-term goal of human gene therapy for sickle cell disease" was in reach, and that the breakthrough would merely consist of "constructing optimally safe and efficient retroviral packaging lines as well as retroviral vectors containing the human beta-globin gene." The cure was close, they promised. "Success in treating disorders of human hemoglobin only awaits additional technical advances for increasing the efficiency of gene transfer and the level of gene expression."[88] A decade later Nathan acknowledged, "Of course we want to do gene therapy, but no one has a gene therapy system that produces enough hemoglobin consistently."[89] Among blood diseases, other disorders like hemophilia and Fanconi's anemia seemed more likely targets for gene therapy. Pessimistically, Nathan concluded that the likelihood of gene therapy in SCD was remote; it was "possibly a dream." A 1996 study found that "most of the work in gene therapy for single-gene inherited disease has focused on cystic fibrosis . . . , the most common autosomal recessive disease in Caucasians in the United States." By the end of 1997, before gene therapy fell on truly hard times, Nathan's pessimism seemed to be another indicator of SCD patients' disadvantages. There were almost twenty gene therapy clinical trials in cystic fibrosis but, not surprisingly, none in sickle cell disease.[90]

These diverse discussions about therapeutic futures reflected different pasts and different cultural investments. Most notably, the issue of community identity had long been part of the discussion of sickle cell disease. As with Tay-Sachs disease, discussions about what constituted appropriate therapy for SCD were inseparable from cultural concerns—community self-determination, cultural attitudes toward therapy, and socioeconomic status. By contrast, with cystic fibrosis, the "Caucasian genetic disease," issues of community identity were largely effaced under the vague rubric of "whiteness," which (as we argue in the previous chapter) suggested a more diffuse sense of belonging, without the specific cultural meanings and stereotypes associated with Jewish or black identity in America. The purveyors of CF gene therapy might allude to the *whiteness* of the disease, but their concern was to sell the idea of gene therapy (the risky venture) in the broadest possible market. For them, the reference was more a rhetorical strategy than a response to patients, families, and community politics. For sickle cell researchers and physicians, the racial experiences of patients have been considerably more than a convenient and vague allusion. For practitioners and patients, pain and infection management, the unfulfilled dream of desickling agents, and the gamble inherent in BMT were routinely racialized —and made to resonate with social and political meanings. The history of race and therapy played a vital role whenever physicians, patients, and families considered the promise and the dangers of unproven therapeutic innovation.

As the hematologist Hugh Chaplin wrote in his 2003 memoir, bone marrow transplantation was merely the latest example of "unrealistic expectations and unnecessary heartbreak," with extraordinary promise on one side and peril on the other.[91] Hematologists have grappled with the false promises of unbridled optimism since before the age of genetic medicine. They have also confronted a wide range of ethical, social, and economic questions surrounding diverse therapeutic options. In many respects, that history was more than a dress rehearsal for the present; it was also an active part of an ongoing, evolving experience, shaping the cautious evaluation of genetic medicine. Given this historical trajectory of race and medical innovation, there is every reason to believe that this experience will color assessments about the grand possibility of genetic transformation for decades to come.

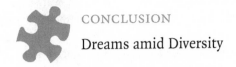

From the rise of antibiotics to the advent of bone marrow transplantation to the age of gene therapy, the promise of a coming therapeutic revolution has always had its allure. "Twenty years from now, gene therapy will have revolutionized the practice of medicine," promised W. French Anderson in 1996. Francis Collins, head of the National Human Genome Project and co-discoverer of the cystic fibrosis gene, also endorsed this perspective, saying in 1990 that research on CF "gives credence to the idea that gene therapy will find a significant place in the therapeutic armamentarium."[1] Such pronouncements captured much about the cultural politics of the time. Boosters of genetic medicine seized upon a disease like CF because it sat at the intersection of scientific discovery, business innovation, and medical practice. For a time in the early 1990s the idea of CF gene therapy embodied the hope of an imminent breakthrough in genetic medicine.

Why have such promises of breakthrough treatment played out so differently from one disease to the next? The answer, it seems, revolves around which America one inhabits. Vastly different situations, cultural sensibilities, and expectations have been at work over the years, shaping the experiences of patients and shaping attitudes about particular diseases, about the people suffering from them, and about the promise of medical breakthrough itself. For some—notably, people with sickle cell disease—modern therapy has been a roller-coaster ride, a mix of significant gains and unfulfilled hype. For others, frustration with incremental progress has been a key motif. As we saw in the cystic fibrosis story, a sense of frustrating progress could nurture a hope for imminent breakthroughs, however unrealistic. And in Tay-Sachs disease, attitudes about inevitable decline and loss overshadowed conventional therapeutic expectations and shifted the focus toward innovations in prevention. These diverse attitudes about therapy have been shaped by many factors: the disease experience itself, the broader cultural image of the disorder, the efforts of physicians and entrepreneurs to shape public thinking, and the ideals about the groups (Jewish and African-American minority groups, majority Anglo-Americans) who became closely associated with each disease. To be sure, the politics of race and ethnicity has been one factor complicating the story of innovation.

SELLING THE DREAM: RACE, ETHNICITY, AND THE PROMISE OF GENETIC INNOVATION

What should a multicultural society do when some in that society are willing to take measures to prevent the birth of people with treatable diseases (like cystic fibrosis or sickle cell disease) while others consider those measures extreme? As we saw in chapter 1, discussions about the prevention and potential cure of Tay-Sachs disease impinged directly on questions of Jewish self-preservation while also highlighting broader questions about minority status and genetic medicine in the United States. As more and more diseases are traced to specific genes, and as more and more Americans learn that they may carry the gene for one ailment or another and may pass the malady on to their offspring, such dilemmas will become more common. And as several scholars have observed, "The genetic revolution . . . will not benefit all equally, and some may in fact be greatly disadvantaged by particular applications of genetic science."[2] This problem was at the heart of the debate over the Dor Yeshorim, that unique system of "genetic matchmaking" that emerged among Ultra-Orthodox Jews in the 1980s to combat Tay-Sachs disease and sought in 1990s to extend its program of testing and prevention to cystic fibrosis. "Every single human being, you and me too, we have some genetic risks for our children," geneticist Michael Kaback had commented in 1993, "whether it's cancer, early heart disease, or certain types of mental illness. I don't know where this stops, or who makes the decision where it stops."[3] The comment reveals a quandary in genetic medicine: Should limits be placed on how any group might use genetic knowledge to preserve its distinctive identity and the health of its people amid powerful pressures toward assimilation? This problem, which began as a health concern for Ultra-Orthodox Jews, a tiny minority group in America, would reverberate beyond the boundaries of the synagogue and this insular community.

The plans of the Dor Yeshorim's architects conflicted with the growing promise of gene therapy in cystic fibrosis, and in that tension we see another kind of cultural politics at work—one that extends well beyond the specifics of Ultra-Orthodox Jews in America and points to deeper tensions between minority and majority sensibilities about religious faith, secular life, profit-making, and hope for the future. The grand promise of cure was emerging out of an enduring American faith in progress. It was a faith nurtured by American mainstream culture and its powerful belief that high risks would bring great rewards. From the origins of the nation and indeed into the twenty-first century, these cultural commitments have been deeply informed by Anglo-American Protestant sensibilities about capital accumulation, risk-taking, and the pursuit of profit. As Max Weber noted long ago, "In the United States, the pursuit of wealth, stripped of its religious and ethical meaning, tends to become associated with purely mundane passions, which often actually give it the character of sport."[4] Faith in the market is central to explaining why so many Americans—Jesse Gelsinger among them—could buy into the exuberant therapeutic promises of gene therapy. Of course, many remained skeptical of these promises as well. The culture of hype surrounding breakthrough cures is fundamentally American, and it reflects a kind of faith that is deeply intertwined with American cultural ideals. Yet the hype has evoked a range of different social responses. These different responses—which are at the heart of this book—must also be understood in cultural terms.

Why are some Americans skeptical of the promises—of high risks, rapid rewards, and coming therapeutic breakthroughs—while others are quick to invest in the gamble? The story of sickle cell disease, and particularly the debate over pain management and bone marrow transplantation, presents a disturbing portrait of America, one in which basic health and social services are hard to obtain, in which skepticism about the motives of patients is rampant, and in which high-stakes gambles like BMT are promoted as remedies for a profoundly troubling situation. Over the course of the last century, American sickle cell patients faced a life of recurrent pain in a culture that was not only skeptical of their suffering but also limited access to the drugs to alleviate pain.[5] Debates about the wisdom and ethics of promoting BMT in sickle cell disease also flared up when its adherents insisted that a 10 percent risk of mortality was acceptable. "Some physicians would demand that marrow grafting have almost a zero risk before it should be undertaken in sickle cell disease," wrote BMT pioneer E. Donnall Thomas in 1991. "I think that is an excessive requirement."[6] A troubling innovation for a painful chronic disease prevalent among African Americans, BMT amounted to a high-stakes lottery in which death and cure were both real options—a metaphor for the cultural politics of ethnicity, race, and innovation in our time.

Over the decades many of these therapeutic dramas contained obvious racial and ethnic narratives—stories of struggle, pain, and survival, as in the case of sickle cell disease and Tay-Sachs. In other cases (like that of cystic fibrosis), issues of race flared to the surface only sporadically and unevenly over time. However, the significance of the occasional appearance of race in discussions about CF should not be underestimated. Even though it is often invisible, the idea of whiteness remains a powerful force in American culture, able to be invoked from time to time to mobilize a wide array of public sentiments. When author Frank Deford explained in the early 1980s that CF was "the white version of sickle cell disease," he was pointing to the sense of black ownership that had encircled SCD and was thereby calling for a larger amalgam of ethnic groups spanning the American spectrum to align themselves with the majority cultural ideals and embrace CF as their own malady.[7] This small gesture showed, in the choice of a single term, the ways in which whiteness itself (as well as ideas about black and Jewish identity) could make use of disease symbolically, to forge a unitary identity and to highlight difference from others.

The Dor Yeshorim's plan for managing TSD and CF, the dilemma of bone marrow transplantation in SCD, and the rise and fall of gene therapy in CF raise profound ethical and cultural questions—a fact that the major actors in these dramas, from Michael Kaback to Francis Collins to E. Donnall Thomas, have acknowledged. How heavily should we rely on the profit motive to shape the future of medicine and society? What level of risk should come with new medicines, and who should bear those risks? What limits should be placed on how individuals shape their genetic destiny? Thus, in these unfolding stories of disease, the pursuit of innovative therapies and drugs became microcosms of broader cultural concerns. As scholar Carl Elliott has noted recently, questions about enhancement through medical treatments reveal where American medicine meets the American dream.[8]

Perhaps the most troubling question is how to evaluate diverse and often overblown claims about breakthrough medicine. Relentlessly marketed in the heyday of gene therapy was the promise that medical science stood on the threshold of an era that would soon produce dramatic lifesaving cures, if not a virtual elimination of disease. In 1993, for example, experts in the scientific and lay press spoke glowingly of the possibilities: "Gene Therapy on Newborn Sets Medical Precedent," "Gene Therapy May Save Kids," "Heading off Genetic Diseases in their Infancy," "A Cure of Cystic Fibrosis? Rainbow [Children's Hospital] Cheers New Gene Therapy."[9] It was a notion of imminent transformation buoyed by a longstanding dream of scientific rationality; it was a powerful hope vaguely aligned with the general idea of progress; and it was an ideal of medical and human development that gained increasing power in the late twentieth century. The dream of cure has been deeply imbued with cultural values: hope for the future, the power of capitalism to deliver better lives for its citizens, the notion of an ever-unfolding modernity. The dream of genetic medicine, "bottling the stuff of dreams," has certainly been a part of this larger ideal; and some of its more grandiose claims are not far removed from the unrealistic idea that someday, in the not-too-distant future, there will be no disease at all.[10] Seldom have these powerful ideals been scrutinized. From time to time, a few notes of caution might appear in the headlines: "Genetic Research Escalates—But Locating Flaws Can Be a Long Way from Curing Disease," noted one Seattle newspaper. The London Guardian suggested that ominous shadow loomed around genetic innovation: "Code of Conduct: The So-Called Homosexual Gene Highlights the Dramatic Advance in DNA Research. It Can Save Lives and Alleviate Suffering but It Also Poses Huge Ethical Problems."[11] But even with these cautions, the media reveled in the possibilities of transformation and the likelihood that "inherited diseases like sickle cell anemia and hemophilia might be cured in newborns . . . while adult diseases like cancer and AIDS" might be next in line to benefit.[12] In the history of disease—and, as we have seen, in the histories of TSD, CF, and SCD—this vision of standing "on the threshold" has emerged repeatedly, nurtured by innovators and entrepreneurs and intertwined with the hopes, ideals, and fears of different patient groups and medical communities in ways that are uplifting but also deeply troubling.

The dream of imminent transformation is an integral part of the ideology of the modern medical sciences, of which genetic medicine is a part. There is ample evidence in the history of medicine—for example, in the role of insulin and penicillin in diabetes or in the preventive power of the polio vaccine—to suggest that this dream is both rational and legitimate. Unquestionably, the story of insulin's discovery in the 1920s, its extensive manufacture, and its role in saving the lives of countless patients with diabetes speaks volumes about the dream. Yet the advent of insulin and the polio vaccine also took many decades to play out; and, more important, the actual impact of these breakthroughs on disease and society has been multifaceted. As historian Chris Feudtner has shown, breakthroughs in diabetes care (from insulin in the 1920s to penicillin in the 1940s) allowed patients to live longer, but it also created an entirely new category of person: a chronic diabetes patient who would come to develop long-term complications from life with the disease. Later breakthroughs such as kidney dialysis would address some of these complications, and new questions would emerge about who would cover the costs of these expensive therapeutic interventions. The scientific transmutation of diabetes has made the disease far more prevalent than it was one hundred years ago, and since the 1970s the advent of legislation mandating Medicare payment for dialysis for people with end-stage renal disease (many of them diabetics) has transformed the story of scientific innovation into a story of social justice.[13] Once it was established, this new federal entitlement prompted new questions about the extent to which society should cover the costs of putting innovative care within the reach of all its citizens. Viewed through the historical lens, then, the dream of breakthroughs becomes more socially complex—for transforming dream into lived reality involves political negotiations, competition for resources, and investments of many kinds.

The recent histories of Tay-Sachs disease, cystic fibrosis, and sickle cell disease unearth often hidden dimensions of the promise of breakthrough medicine: the conflict between the cultural allure of the idea of imminent transformation and the realities of what can be delivered to patients; the unintended consequences of experimentation and innovation; and the ways in which scientists, business interests, and social commentators capitalize on this cultural motif in order to draw attention to their respective enterprises, even when their ventures are speculative in the extreme.

It remains to be seen what kind of future the genetics revolution holds for us. To date, the revolution has most transformed society in the areas of diagnosis and prevention. Therapy continues to be a vexing challenge. If the promise of breakthrough cures has often been unrealized, a large part of the problem is rooted in the stubborn asymmetries between scientific and technological models of disease and how bodies actually work. The idea of an adenovirus that transports "good" DNA to the cells in a patient's lungs which then repairs the functioning of the diseased cells is both elegant and naïve. On one hand, there remains something alluring in this simple dream of curing disease, precisely because the dream so radically oversimplifies or stereotypes the complexities of the body itself. On the other hand, the human body is complex and has shown resistance over the years to simplistic manipulation. The logic of the adenovirus as a DNA delivery vehicle did not account for the realities of inflammation that would be caused by the vector. The logic of enzyme replacement did not, at first, reckon on the blood-brain barrier as a powerful impediment. And the logic of bone marrow transplantation, as presented in the headlines, rarely took note of the realities of graft-versus-host-disease. The popular dream of breakthrough medicine seldom dwells on such problems; such worrisome matters do not make the headlines, for they do not capture the public or scientific imagination. Nonetheless, these problems represent the true face of breakthrough medicine, in all its paradoxical wonder and its social and ethical complexity.

The dream of breakthrough medicine often founders when confronted with another asymmetry: between the scientific logic of producing new therapies and the social logic of how the marketplace determines who gains access to those innovations. Throughout the 1990s it became increasingly clear that genetic medicine was not merely a benevolent enterprise dedicated to curing the sick people of the world but also a growing financial enterprise operating according to the edicts of the marketplace. Headlines, once again, told the story: "Worcester Firm a Step Closer to Finding a Gene Therapy: Emerging Business," "A Market That Could Spiral: The Commercial Opportunities of Gene Therapy Are Growing by the Minute," and "Biotech Startup Gets Genentech's Backing: South [San Francisco] Firm to Take 20% Stake in [Gene Therapy Company] GenVec."[14] Clinical experiments were means toward a financial end; one such end was attracting investors with a steady stream of good news, bringing a promising product ever-closer to the market. In this sense the promise of genetic medicine took many of its meanings from the broader business culture of the 1990s and from the strategizing of a new type of researcher/entrepreneur, which was further blurring the lines between innovation for profit and patient care. Not surprisingly, the failures of gene therapy in later years would draw increasing public attention to this profit-seeking aspect of the enterprise and to the ways in which ostensibly benevolent experiments were shaped, clouded, and compromised by the search for profit. But even had it been a success, and had the promised cures emerged from the research process as in the story of Gaucher's disease and enzyme replacement therapy, these same forces would have continued to shape the cost and accessibility of innovative treatments.

In their efforts to convince others of the far-reaching value of medical innovations like gene therapy, those selling the dream insisted that the ripples of innovation would span the nation—that is, the benefits would accrue to a wide range of racial and ethnic groups. As one article suggested in the 1990s, "Gene therapy offers promise in future for sickle cell anemia," while others repeatedly noted that cystic fibrosis was the most common genetic disease among Caucasians.[15] Such references were never accidental. Society places a great deal of stock in what scientists tell us about race and ethnicity, looking to these experts to tell us about the biological bases of our cultural differences. Genetic analysis and population studies of Tay-Sachs disease, for example, told the story of its links to Ashkenazic Jewish populations and also to populations like French Canadians and Louisiana Cajuns. Sickle cell disease taught about its links to malaria and African survival.

The notion of cystic fibrosis as an important Caucasian disease became the focus of wide-ranging speculation about European and Caucasian history and identity, for the CF gene seemed to span eons from the age of early man to the present.[16] In the 1990s, studies of the DF508 gene, the most common among the more than two hundred mutations responsible for CF, became a key reference point for speculation and myth-making about European identity.

Despite the apparent links between disease and racial identity, the specifics of these links proved to be malleable and subject to change. Indeed, the idea of "race" carried strikingly different meanings in each disease. For example, as we saw in chapter 2, when one cystic fibrosis expert was faced with the need to lobby Congress for research funds in 1972, at a time when "white" diseases might not have gained a sympathetic hearing, he comfortably asserted the panethnic nature of CF. When researchers in the 1990s spoke of CF as a "white" disease, they were also attempting to evoke a set of shared cultural assumptions—not about panethnicity but about the particular benefits that might accrue from genetic innovation for that majority of Americans who identified themselves as white. Such diseases—from Tay-Sachs to sickle cell disease to cystic fibrosis—could be called upon at various times to do a kind of cultural heavy lifting, to signal the broad scope and significance of scientific work, to ensure cultural and financial investments in a promising scientific and medical enterprise.

By the late 1990s and into the first years of the twenty-first century, the gene therapy news had taken a turn for the worse. Again, the headlines in 2004 told of new problems with the dream: "FDA Suspends Gene Therapy Work," "Why Gene Therapy Still Hasn't Produced Major Breakthroughs," "Gene Genie Stays in Bottle," "Gene Therapy Is Just an Expensive Myth, Claims Scientist."[17] The enterprise deflated precipitously beginning in the late 1990s, its promise sapped by experimental failures, by the deaths of patients, by new concerns about cancer risk, and by the bursting of the inflated biotechnology bubble. Yet if the dream of curative gene therapy appears out of reach, the allure of genetic medicine remains strong.

"THE KING IS DEAD, LONG LIVE THE KING":
FROM GENE THERAPY TO PHARMACOGENOMICS

At precisely the time when gene therapy was being declared moribund, a new promise was emerging: the dream of pharmacogenomics, the idea of targeting drugs to the specific genetic makeup of patients in order to deliver cures that more precisely matched the workings of their individual bodies. As so often happens in medicine, in late 2004 an old drug resurfaced with novel uses. Five years earlier the Food and Drug Administration had rejected the drug BiDil for use in the "general population," but the company producing the drug sought and received permission from the FDA in 2001 to test the drug in African-American heart-failure patients.

The story of BiDil evoked many of the themes that shadowed the therapeutic histories of Tay-Sachs disease, cystic fibrosis, and sickle cell disease: the roller-coaster ride of therapy, the tensions between faith in breakthroughs and skepticism about grand promises. In this second round of clinical trials, BiDil proved effective for treating heart failure in roughly one thousand African Americans, whose heart disease tended to be more severe than that found in the "general," predominantly white, population of patients with heart disease. Trials were immediately halted, the drug was declared a success, and media accounts voiced both wonder and skepticism about the findings. One journalist asked, "Is it good science—or shrewd marketing?" No one could reliably say why the drug had worked in this study or whether race and ethnicity were indeed key factors in the its effectiveness; and although there was no effort to study the genes or genetic features of the patients per se, the story was quickly framed as "the leading edge of race-based pharmacogenomics."[18] The story sent a diverse range of biological and economic messages. As Jonathan Katz remarked, "BiDil became an ethnic drug through the interventions of law and commerce as much as through medical understanding of biological differences that correlate with racial groups."[19] Indeed, from the start of the clinical trial the Massachusetts-based company, NitroMed, argued that the drug's ability to remedy nitric-oxide deficiency (which NitroMed argued was more common in black heart-failure patients than in others) "might make it especially suited" for black patients.[20] The company's president and chief executive, Dr. Loberg, noted that the market for the drug was quite large since "there were about 750,000 blacks with heart failure . . . and if all of them used the drug, sales could reach $1 billion a year."[21]

Beneath the catchy and simplistic headlines suggesting that this was an instance in which genetics, disease, race, and ethnicity came together, a much more complicated story emerged; indeed, many different and conflicted notions about race biology remained unreconciled in the BiDil story. "What we're talking about is a selective prevalence of the mechanism," said Dr. Anne Taylor, the lead researcher in the clinical trial. "It doesn't mean that every member of that group possesses this mechanism [of drug action]." Or, as another physician put it, "It doesn't mean that it's unique to that group."[22] Much of the controversy surrounding "the black pill" revolved around the question of who benefits and profits from this kind of targeted research and marketing. One cardiologist worried that "approving and marketing a drug to one group only could hurt other patients who might have benefited from the same treatment."[23] Another commentator turned this line of inquiry back onto the socially constructed nature of "blackness" itself, asking, "Does the drug work more effectively on dark-skinned blacks than light-skinned, vanilla-colored vs. caramel, deep-chocolate-colored vs. high yellow? What level of black blood, DNA or gradation of complexion must African Americans have to be good candidates to receive the drug and have it work effectively?"[24] Still another observer, reaching for compromise, noted, "We need not shy away from the potential benefits of race-conscious therapeutics, but we should manage its downside risks." What was needed was "greater awareness among physicians and the public that race is at best a placeholder for other predispositions, and not a biologic verity."[25] Such questions highlighted, of course, the intense skepticism greeting the BiDil claims as well as the complex matrix of attitudes about skin color, racial identity, fairness, and marketing hype that have historically shadowed discussions about race, genetics, and medicine.

That one promise of genetic breakthrough should emerge just as another is collapsing should not surprise us. Maintaining faith in innovation, especially amid controversy, is a complex cultural process that resembles other patterns for shoring up hope, trust, and faith in authority. In former times, and still today, the sovereignty of the king was assured by his two bodies: one corporeal, the other symbolic. His corporeal body might expire, but the king never perished, for he was always to be replaced by another. Thus was the principle of succession supported, assuring order in times of crisis. In the age of modern biomedicine, the authority of therapeutic innovation depends in no small part on a similar logic of succession: a powerful cultural belief in the sick body's capacity to be transformed by the reigning cure of the day, if not through gene therapy, as promised in the 1990s, then through pharmacogenomics in the years to come. Indeed, as we have seen in the stories of Tay-Sachs disease, cystic fibrosis, and sickle cell disease, this pattern is part of the long and fascinating history of therapeutic promises and genetic developments. It is a recurring theme of the past half-century: when one breakthrough fails to play out as predicted or has unwelcome consequences, another will emerge to take its place or to resolve the mess created in the wake.

Nor should it surprise us that questions of race and ethnicity are so often at the forefront of breakthrough medicine. For researchers and reporters alike, the act of linking race to stories of innovation dramatizes and broadens the cultural significance of the innovation. In this context, grand claims about the future of therapy can easily segue into a different set of discussions—about justice, fairness, the pursuit of equality, self-determination, and the effort to nurture and maintain identity in modern America. These issues, we argue, are often obscured by the headlines, by the hype associated with breakthrough medicine. Beneath the headlines lies a more complex story, a story about suffering and faith, about unevenness in the distribution of risks and rewards, about the marketing of dreams, about how diverse Americans embrace innovation, and about how each of us grapples in our own way with the promise of a better life to come.

NOTES

INTRODUCTION. ETHNIC SYMBOLS IN CONFLICTED TIMES

1 The interaction between race, ethnicity, and innovation spawned many controversies over the years. A complete list would be too long to provide here. Some of the most prominent examples include the Tuskegee experiment on the impact of untreated syphilis in African-American Southern men dating from the 1930s to the early 1970s; Nazi-era experimentation on Jews, Gypsies, and others; the field trials testing the birth control pill in Puerto Rico beginning in the mid-1950s; the development and testing of AIDS drugs and vaccines in the developing world; and the recent history of the Human Genome Diversity Project. For more on these topics, see James Jones, *Bad Blood: The Tuskegee Syphilis Experiment* (New York: Free Press, 1981); Annette Ramirez and Conrad Seipp, *Colonialism, Catholicism, and Contraception* (Chapel Hill: University of North Carolina Press, 1983); Benno Muller-Hill, *Murderous Science: Elimination by Scientific Selection of Jews, Gypsies, and Others, Germany, 1933–1945*, trans. G. Fraser (Cold Spring Harbor: Cold Spring Harbor Laboratory Press, 1998); Nicolas Nattrass, *The Moral Economy of AIDS in South Africa* (New York: Cambridge University Press, 2003); and Jenny Reardon, *Race to the Finish: Identity and Governance in the Age of Genomics* (Princeton: Princeton University Press, 2004). See also S. J. Gould, *The Mismeasure of Man* (New York: W. W. Norton, 1981).

2 David Suzuki and Peter Knudtson, *Genethics: The Clash between the New Genetics and Human Values* (Cambridge, Mass.: Harvard University Press, 1989); Philip Kitcher, *The Lives to Come: The Genetic Revolution and Human Possibilities* (New York: Simon and Schuster, 1996); Daniel Kevles and Leroy Hood, eds., *The Code of Codes: Scientific and Social Issues in the Human Genome Project* (Cambridge, Mass.: Harvard University Press, 1992); and the essays in Timothy Murphy and Marc Lappe, eds., *Justice and the Human Genome Project* (Berkeley and Los Angeles: University of California Press, 1994), in particular Arthur Caplan, "Handle with Care: Race, Class and Genetics," Norman Daniels, "The Genome Project, Individual Difference, and Just Health Care," Leonard Fleck, "Just Genetics: A Problem Agenda," and Marc Lappe, "Justice and the Limitations of Genetic Knowledge."

3 Lawrence Fisher, "Bottling the Stuff of Dreams: Gains in Gene Therapy Encourage the Industry," *New York Times*, 1 June 1995, D1; Robert Schulman et al., "The Gene Doctors: Scientists Are on the Verge of Curing Life's Cruelest Diseases," *Business Week*, 18 November 1985, 76–80.

4 The scholarly literature on the social and cultural aspects of genetic disease, genetic medicine (screening, therapy, and risks), and public perceptions of genetics has grown dramatically in recent years, and includes works by anthropologists, sociologists, historians, and philosophers. See, for example, M. Susan Lindee, *Moments of Truth in Genetic Medicine* (Baltimore: Johns Hopkins University Press, 2005); Troy Duster, *Backdoor to Eugenics*, 2d ed. (New York: Routledge, 2003); Jenny Reardon, *Race to the Finish: Identity and Governance in the Age of Genomics* (Princeton: Princeton University Press, 2005); Paul Rabinow, *French DNA: Trouble in Purgatory* (Chicago: University of Chicago Press, 1999); Paul Martin, "Genes as Drugs: The Social Shaping of Gene Therapy and the Reconstruction of Genetic Disease," *Sociology of Health and Illness* 21 (1999): 517–38; Alan Stockdale, "Waiting for the Cure: Mapping the Social Relations of Human Gene Therapy Research," *Sociology of Health and Illness* 21 (1999): 579–96; Dorothy Nelkin and M. Susan Lindee, *The DNA Mystique: The Gene as Cultural Icon* (New York: W. H. Freeman, 1995); Celeste Michelle Condit, *The Meanings of the Gene: Public Debates about Human Heredity* (Madison: University of Wisconsin Press, 1999); Michael Ruse, "Does Genetic Counselling Really Raise the Quality of Life?" in *Is Science Sexist? and Other Problems in the Biomedical Sciences* (Boston: D. Reidel, 1981), 130–57; Rayna Rapp, *Testing Women, Testing the Fetus: The Social Impact of Amniocentesis in America* (New York: Routledge, 1999); Rayna Rapp, "Risky Business: Genetic Counseling in a Shifting World," in *Articulating Hidden Histories*, ed. Jane Schneider and Rayna Rapp (Berkeley and Los Angeles: University of California Press, 1995), 175–89; Carlos Novas and Nikolas Rose, "Genetic Risk and the Birth of the Somatic Individual," *Economy and Society* 29 (November 2000): 485–513; Kaja Finkler, "Illusions of Controlling the Future: Risk and Genetic Inheritance," *Anthropology and Medicine* 10 (2003): 51–70; and Karen-Sue Taussig, Rayna Rapp, and Deborah Heath, "Flexible Eugenics: Technologies of the Self in the Age of Genetics," in *Genetic Nature/Culture: Anthropology and Science beyond the Two-Culture Divide*, ed. Alan H. Goodman, Deborah Heath, and M. Susan Lindee (Berkeley and Los Angeles: University of California Press, 2003), 51–76. On medi-

cal genetics and religious, ethnic, and national identity, see Karen-Sue Taussig, "Calvinism and Chromosomes: Religion, the Geographical Imaginary, and Medical Genetics in the Netherlands," *Science as Culture* 6 (1997): 495–524, and Susan Martha Kahn, *Reproducing Jews: A Cultural Account of Assisted Conception in Israel* (Durham: Duke University Press, 2000).

The literature on the cultural and social aspects of Tay-Sachs disease, cystic fibrosis, and sickle cell disease is also significant. For historical comparisons of the three disorders, see Howard Markel, "Scientific Advances and Social Risks: Historical Perspectives of Genetic Screening Programs for Sickle Cell Disease, Tay-Sachs Disease, Neural Tube Defects, and Down Syndrome, 1970–1997," in *Promoting Safe and Effective Genetic Testing in the United States: Final Report of the Task Force on Genetic Testing*, ed. Neil Holtzman and Michael Watson (Baltimore: Johns Hopkins University Press, 1998), 161–76, and Keith Wailoo, "Inventing the Heterozygote: Molecular Biology, Racial Identity, and the Narratives of Sickle-Cell Disease, Tay-Sachs, and Cystic Fibrosis," in *Race, Nature, and the Politics of Difference*, ed. Donald Moore, Jake Kosek, and Anand Pandian (Durham: Duke University Press, 2003), 235–53. On cystic fibrosis, see Lene Koch and Dirk Stemerding, "The Sociology of Entrenchment—A Cystic Fibrosis Test for Everyone," *Social Science and Medicine* 39 (1994): 1211–20; Alan Stockdale, "Conflicting Perspectives: Coping with Cystic Fibrosis in the Age of Molecular Medicine," Ph.D. diss., Brandeis University, 1997; Anne Kerr, "(Re)Constructing Genetic Disease: The Clinical Continuum between Cystic Fibrosis and Male Infertility," *Social Studies of Science* 30 (2000): 847–94; and Adam M. Hedgecoe, "Expansion and Uncertainty: Cystic Fibrosis, Classification and Genetics," *Sociology of Health and Illness* 25 (January 2003): 50–70. On sickle cell disease, see Keith Wailoo, *Drawing Blood: Technology and Disease Identity in Twentieth-Century America* (Baltimore: Johns Hopkins University Press, 1997); Melbourne Tapper, *In the Blood: Sickle Cell Anemia and the Politics of Race* (Philadelphia: University of Pennsylvania Press, 1999); Keith Wailoo, *Dying in the City of the Blues: Sickle Cell Anemia and the Politics of Race* (Chapel Hill: University of North Carolina Press, 2001); Duana Fullwiley, "Life, Ethics, and Sickle Cell Anemia: A Single Gene Disorder in a Contingent World," Ph.D. diss., University of California Berkeley/University of California San Francisco, 2002; Duana Fullwiley, "Discriminate Biopower and Everyday Biopolitics: Views on

Sickle Cell Testing in Dakar," *Medical Anthropology* 23 (April/June 2004): 157–95; and Carolyn Moxley Rouse, "Paradigms and Politics: Shaping Health Care Access for Sickle Cell Patients through the Discursive Regimes of Biomedicine," *Culture, Medicine, and Psychiatry* 28 (2004): 369–99.

5 Linus Pauling, "Reflections on a New Biology: Foreword," *UCLA Law Review* 15 (1968): 269; Gina Kolata, "Nightmare or the Dream of a New Era in Genetics?" *New York Times*, 7 December 1993, A1.

6 Ellen Lee, "On the Front Lines against Cystic Fibrosis," *Atlanta Journal and Constitution*, 23 August 1998, C4. Also Michael Kernan, "A Death in the Family: Frank Deford's Poignant Goodbye to His Daughter," *Washington Post*, 27 October 1983, D1.

7 TSD, CF, and SCD are all autosomal recessive traits, which means that they each result from the inheritance of two defective traits (or genes), one from each parent. Thus, when both parents are carriers of the faulty genetic trait, any child they conceive has a 25 percent chance of being free of the trait, a 50 percent chance of inheriting the trait, and a 25 percent chance of inheriting the disease itself (a double dose of the trait).

8 Madeleine Goodman and Lenn Goodman, "The Overselling of Genetic Anxiety," *Hastings Center Report*, October 1982, 20–27.

9 Particularly useful studies of these three childhood diseases (and child health in general) include Frank Deford, *Alex: The Life of a Child* (New York: Viking, 1983); Sydney Halpern, *American Pediatrics: The Social Dynamics of Professionalism, 1880–1980* (Berkeley and Los Angeles: University of California Press, 1988); *Suffer the Children: The Story of Thalidomide* (New York: Viking Press, 1979); Stuart Edelstein, *The Sickled Cell: From Myths to Molecules* (Cambridge, Mass.: Harvard University Press, 1986); Bruce Shapiro and Ralph Heussner, *A Parent's Guide to Cystic Fibrosis* (Minneapolis: University of Minnesota Press, 1991); and Michael Kaback, ed., *Tay-Sachs Disease: Screening and Prevention* (New York: Alan R. Liss, 1977).

10 Hugh Chaplin, *Lenabell: A Doctor's Memoir of a Remarkable Woman's Eighty Year Battle with Sickle Cell Disease* (Philadelphia: Xlibris, 2003); Andrew Purvis, "Laying Siege to a Deadly Gene: Thanks to Series of Breakthroughs, Doctors Are Closing in on a Cure for Cystic Fibrosis," *Time*, 24 February 1992, 60.

11 Barbara Culliton, "Cooley's Anemia: Special Treatment for Another

Ethnic Disease," *Science* 178 (10 November 1972): 590–93; Kernan, "A Death in the Family," D1.

12 Herbert J. Gans, "Symbolic Ethnicity: The Future of Ethnic Groups and Cultures in America," in *On the Making of Americans: Essays in Honor of David Riesman*, ed. Herbert Gans et al. (Philadelphia: University of Pennsylvania Press, 1979), 193; reprinted in Werner Sollors, ed., *Theories of Ethnicity: A Classical Reader* (Washington Square, N.Y.: New York University Press, 1996), 425.

13 On one hand, modern genetic information about diseases like TSD, CF, and SCD have reinforced ideas about fundamental biological differences. On the other hand, believers in the new genetics insist that these differences are not real — that careful and thorough study of the role of a wider range of genes across human populations will eventually force a radical rethinking of time-worn notions of race, ethnicity, and group identity. They argue that the distribution of genes across populations will reveal profound linkages across groups, suggesting that medicine will take its future cues from our genes rather than from our skin color or ethnic affiliations. In this new world, it is said, we may come to see that genetic risks carried by any single individual may make that person closer kin with another individual carrying those same genetic risks, regardless of their race or ethnicity. A new biological reality may well come to supplant the older one, at least in the realm of scientific research and medicine. This is one perspective on race, biology, and identity taking shape today, for example, in the new field of pharmacogenomics.

14 Diane Paul, "Eugenic Origins of Medical Genetics," in *The Politics of Heredity: Essays on Eugenics, Biomedicine, and the Nature-Nurture Debate* (Albany: SUNY Press, 1998), 149, quoting Frederick Osborn, *The Future of Human Heredity* (New York: Harper and Brothers, 1968), 25.

15 Richard Lewontin, *Biology as Ideology: The Doctrine of DNA* (New York: Perennial, 1993); Edward Yoxen, "Constructing Genetic Diseases," in *The Problem of Medical Knowledge: Examining the Social Construction of Medicine*, ed. P. Wright and A. Treacher (Edinburgh: Edinburgh University Press, 1982), 144–61; Richard Lewontin, *It Ain't Necessarily So: The Dream of the Human Genome and Other Illusions* (New York: New York Review of Books, 2001); Troy Duster, *Backdoor to Eugenics* (New York: Routledge, 1990).

16 Joseph Graves, *The Emperor's New Clothes: Biological Theories of Race at the*

Millennium (New Brunswick: Rutgers University Press, 2003); Jonathan Marks, *Human Biodiversity: Genes, Race, and History* (New York: Aldine, 1995); Steve Olsen, *Mapping Human History: Genes, Race, and Our Common Origins* (New York: Mariner Books, 2003). Also Karen Brodkin, *How Jews Became White Folks and What That Says about Race in America* (New Brunswick: Rutgers University Press, 1998); Ruth Frankenberg, *White Women, Race Matters: The Social Construction of Whiteness* (Minneapolis: University of Minnesota Press, 1993).

17 Various scholars have pointed out the fabricated nature of Caucasian as a racial concept. As English biologist Thomas Henry Huxley wrote in 1868, "Of all the odd myths that have arisen in the scientific world, the 'Caucasian mystery' invented quite innocently by [Johann Friedrich] Blumenbach [in 1775] is the oddest. A Georgian woman's skull was the handsomest in his collection. Hence it became his model exemplar of human skulls, from which all the others might be regarded as deviations; and out of this, by some strange intellectual hocus-pocus, grew up the notion that the Caucasian man is the prototypic 'Adamic' man." After Huxley wrote, the term *Caucasian* became associated with the origins of the Anglo-Saxon and Aryan races on similarly mythic grounds. Since World War II, the term *Caucasian* has been most frequently used as a synonym for *white*. At every stage in its history, the concept of "Caucasian" has been convoluted and problematic. See Matthew Frye Jacobsen, *Whiteness of a Different Color: European Immigrants and the Alchemy of Race* (Cambridge, Mass.: Harvard University Press, 1998), 1–14, Huxley quotation at 1.

18 Nor should this book be seen as an effort to track the epidemiological history of these maladies—to follow their rising and falling prevalence over time. To be sure, SCD and CF appear to have grown in prevalence over the last half century, while in the last few decades occurrences of TSD—a much rarer disease than the other two—have diminished. SCD is said to occur in 1 in every 400 births to African-American parents; CF is said to occur at a similar rate among white Americans; and TSD has a recorded incidence of 1 per 3,600 births to Ashkenazic Jewish parents. (See also the information on pp. 27, 92, and 133 for carrier frequency and disease incidence.) While the following pages give some insight into shifts in these figures over time, a full epidemiological portrait is well beyond the scope of this book. Indeed, such a history would require the analysis of health statistics that are incom-

plete. Moreover, disease like CF and SCD were widely seen as "great masqueraders" in the 1950s and 1960s, often evading diagnosis simply because they mimicked so many other diseases. Any attempt to reconstruct an epidemiological history would fail, given dramatic historical shifts in the identification of such maladies.

19 Crystal quoted in Natalie Angier, "Cystic Fibrosis: Experiment Hits a Snag," *New York Times*, 22 September 1993, C12; "Waking up Genes: A Flavor Enhancer May Provide the First Treatment for Sickle Cell Anemia," *Time*, 25 January 1993, 23.

20 Steven Epstein, *Impure Science: AIDS, Activism, and the Politics of Knowledge* (Berkeley and Los Angeles: University of California Press, 1998); Laura K. Potts, ed., *Ideology of Breast Cancer: Feminist Perspectives* (New York: Palgrave, 2000); Anne S. Kasper and Susan Ferguson, eds., *Breast Cancer: Society Shapes an Epidemic* (New York: St. Martin's, 2000).

21 The growing influence of genetics has already altered community and family relationships and profoundly influenced our ideas about kinship—a process anthropologist Kaja Finkler calls "the medicalization of kinship." Kaja Finkler, *Experiencing the New Genetics: Family and Kinship on the Medical Frontier* (Philadelphia: University of Pennsylvania Press, 2000). See also Alice Wexler, *Mapping Fate: A Memoir of Family, Risk, and Genetic Research* (New York: Random House, 1995); Rayna Rapp, "Extra Chromosomes and Blue Tulips: Medico-Familial Interpretations," in *Living and Working with the New Medical Technologies*, ed. Margaret Lock, Allan Young, Alberto Cambrosio, and Alan Harwood (New York: Cambridge University Press, 2000), 184–208; Kaja Finkler, "The Kin in the Gene [with Commentaries]," *Current Anthropology* 42 (2001): 235–63; Rayna Rapp, Deborah Heath, and Karen-Sue Taussig, "Genealogical Dis-Ease: Where Hereditary Abnormality, Biomedical Explanation, and Family Responsibility Meet," in *Relative Values: Reconfiguring Kinship Studies*, ed. Sarah Franklin and Susan McKinnon (Durham: Duke University Press, 2001), 384–409; Rayna Rapp, "Cell Life and Death, Child Life and Death: Genomic Horizons, Genetic Diseases, Family Stories," in *Remaking Life and Death: Toward an Anthropology of the Biosciences*, ed. Sarah Franklin and Margaret Lock (Santa Fe: School of American Research Press, 2003), 129–64; and Kaja Finkler, Cécile Skrzynia, and James P. Evans, "The New Genetics and Its Consequences for Family, Kinship, Medicine, and Medical Genetics," *Social Science and Medicine* 57 (August 2003): 403–12.

1 Jane Feldman Paritzky, "Tay-Sachs: The Dreaded Inheritance," *American Journal of Nursing*, March 1985, 262–63.

2 "Denouement and Discussion: Tay Sachs Disease," *American Journal of the Diseases of Children* 146 (June 1992): 768.

3 As Horace Kellen wrote in 1915, "And finally the Jews. Their attitude toward America is different in a fundamental respect from that of other immigrant nationalities. They do not come to the United States from truly native lands . . . They come from lands of sojourn where they have been for ages treated as foreigners . . . Yet, once . . . the Jewish immigrant takes his place in our society a free man and an American, he tends to become all the more a Jew." Horace Kellen, "Democracy versus the Melting Pot: A Study of American Nationality," *Nation*, 18 February 1915, 190–94, and 25 February 1915, 217–20, reprinted in Werner Sollors, ed., *Theories of Ethnicity: A Classical Reader* (Washington Square, N.Y.: New York University Press, 1996), 67–92, at 86–87.

4 Robert Salvayre, Louis Douste-Blazy, and Shimon Gatt, eds., *Lipid Storage Disorders: Biological and Medical Aspects* (New York: Plenum Press, 1987).

5 Karen Bellenir, ed., *Genetic Disorders Sourcebook*, vol. 13 (New York: Ruffner, 1996); see pt. 3, Lysosomal Storage Diseases.

6 Bruno Volk and Larry Schneck, eds., *The Gangliosidoses* (New York: Plenum Press, 1975); Stanley Aronson and Bruno Volk, eds., *Cerebral Sphingolipidoses: A Symposium on Tay-Sachs' Disease and Allied Disorders* (New York: Academic Press, 1962). One author called TSD "the prototype of human sphingolipidoses." Kousaku Ohno, "Molecular Genetics of Beta-N-Acetylhexosaminidase Alpha Subunit Mutations," in *Lipid Storage Disorders*, ed. Salvayre, Douste-Blazy, and Gatt, 215.

7 Paul Edelson, "The Tay-Sachs Disease Screening Program in the U.S. as a Model for the Control of Genetic Disease: An Historical Overview," *Health Matrix* 7 (winter 1997): 125–33; James E. Bowman, "Cultural and Ethnic Differences in Genetic Testing," in *Genetics in the Clinic: Clinical, Ethical, and Social Implications for Primary Care*, ed. Mary Mahowald, Victor McKusick, Angela Scheuerle, and Timothy Aspinwall (St. Louis: Mosby, 2001), 107. See also Michael Kaback, Joyce Lim-Steele, Deepti Dabholkar, David Brown, Nancy Levy, Karen Zeiger, and the International TSD Data Collection Network, "Tay-Sachs Disease—Carrier Screening, Prenatal Diagnosis, and the Molecular Era: An Interna-

tional Perspective, 1970 to 1993," *Journal of the American Medical Association* 270 (17 November 1993): 2307–15. For comparative discussion of CF screening, see U.S. Congress, Office of Technology Assessment, *Cystic Fibrosis and DNA Tests: Implications for Carrier Screening*, OTA-BA-532 (Washington, D.C.: U.S. Government Printing Office, 1992), 256.

8 Nicholas Wade, "Two Scholarly Articles Diverge on Role of Race in Medicine," *New York Times*, 20 March 2003, A30.

9 Rabbi Steven Jacobs, "A Religious Response to Tay-Sachs Disease Screening and Prevention," and Rabbi Edward Tenenbaum, "A Conservative Jewish View of the Tay-Sachs Screening Procedures," both in *Tay-Sachs Disease: Screening and Prevention*, ed. Michael Kaback (New York: Alan R. Liss, 1977), 75–94.

10 See Karen Brodkin, *How Jews Became White Folks and What That Says about Race in America* (New Brunswick: Rutgers University Press, 1998), and Richard Delgado and Jean Stefancic, eds., *Critical White Studies: Looking behind the Mirror* (Philadelphia: Temple University Press, 1997).

11 Gina Kolata, "Using Genetic Tests, Ashkenazi Jews Vanquish a Disease," *New York Times*, 18 February 2003, F1.

12 Quoted in Alison George, "The Rabbi's Dilemma," *New Scientists*, 14 February 2004, 44.

13 Bonnie Friedman, "Tay-Sachs and Other Lipid Storage Diseases," *HSMHA Health Reports* 86 (September 1971): 774. "When such a diagnosis is made, prospective patients have the opportunity to consider therapeutic abortion."

14 Clare Kittredge, "High Tay-Sachs Risk Seen in Franco-Americans," *New Hampshire Weekly*, 19 April 1992, 1.

15 Donna St. George, "The Toll of Tay-Sachs Disease: In Rural Louisiana, the Mystifying Deaths of 'Lazy Babies' Are Solved," *Washington Post*, 8 January 1991, 8. See also J. Michael Kennedy, "A Tragic Legacy," *Los Angeles Times*, 6 November 1990, E1, and John Pope, "Deadly Hereditary Disease Cuts a Swath in Rural LA," *New Orleans Times-Picayune*, 4 October 1990, A1.

16 Quoted in Tim Cornwell, "Jewish Marriage Makers Embrace Testing for Genetic Disease," *London Guardian*, 6 March 1994, 27.

17 Quoted in Gina Kolata, "Nightmare or the Dream of a New Era in Genetics?" *New York Times*, 7 December 1993, A1.

18 W. Tay, "Symmetrical Changes in the Region of the Yellow Spot in Each Eye of an Infant," *Transactions of the Ophthalmological Society (U.K.)*

1 (1881): 55–57; B. Sachs, "On Arrested Cerebral Development with Special Reference to Its Cortical Pathology," *Journal of Nervous and Mental Diseases* 14 (1887): 541; B. Sachs, "A Family Form of Idiocy, Generally Fatal, Associated with Early Blindness," *Journal of Nervous and Mental Diseases* 21 (1896): 475–79. A useful overview of this early history is Michael Kaback, "Tay-Sachs Disease: From Clinical Description to Prospective Control," in *Tay-Sachs Disease*, ed. Kaback, 1–7.

19 Valerie Cowie, "An Inbuilt Tragedy," *Nursing Mirror*, 23 February 1983, 48.

20 Sachs, "Family Form of Idiocy." See also D. Slome, "The Genetic Basis of Amaurotic Family Idiocy," *Journal of Genetics* 27 (1933): 363–72.

21 Quoted in P. R. Evans, "Tay-Sachs Disease: A Centenary," *Archives of Disease in Childhood* 62 (1987): 1056–59, at 1058.

22 Ernst Klenk, "Beitrage zur chemie der lipodosen (3 mitteilung). Niemann-Picksche krankheit und amaurotische idiote," *Hoppe-Seylers Zeitschrift für Physiologische Chemie* 262 (1939–40): 128–43; Ernst Klenk, "Uber die ganglioside des gehirns bei der infantilen amaurotischen idiotie vom typus Tay-Sachs," *Berichte der Deutschen Chemischen Gesellschaft* 75 (1942): 1632–36.

23 Lars Svennerholm, "The Chemical Structure of Normal Human Brain and Tay-Sachs Gangliosides," *Biochemical and Biophysical Research Communications* 9 (1962): 436; Lars Svennerholm, "The Gangliosides," *Journal of Lipid Research* 41 (April 1964): 145–55; Bruno W. Volk, ed. *Tay-Sachs Disease* (New York: Grune and Stratton, 1964); H. G. Hers, *Gastroenterology* 48 (1965): 625. See also R. Ledeen and K. Salsman, "Structure of the Tay-Sachs' Ganglioside, I," *Biochemistry* 4 (1965): 2225–32.

24 Slome, "Genetic Basis of Amaurotic Family Idiocy"; S. M. Aronson, M. P. Valsamis, and B. W. Volk, "Infantile Amaurotic Family Idiocy: Occurrences, Genetic Considerations, and Pathophysiology in the Non-Jewish Infant," *Pediatrics* 26 (1960): 229–42.

25 Roscoe Brady, "Tay-Sachs Disease," *New England Journal of Medicine* 281 (1969): 1243–44, at 1243.

26 Bruno Volk, "Understanding Tay-Sachs Disease: Recent Advances," *Clinical Pediatrics* 5 (November 1966): 653–54; Robert H. Wilkins and Irwin A. Brody, "Tay-Sachs' Disease," *Archives of Neurology* 20 (January 1969): 103.

27 Shintaro Okada and John O'Brien, "Tay-Sachs Disease: Generalized

Absence of a Beta-D-N-acetylhexosaminidase Component," *Science* 165 (15 August 1969): 698–700.

28 John O'Brien, Shintaro Okada, A. Chen, and Dorothy Fillerup, "Tay-Sachs Disease: Detection of Heterozygotes and Homozygotes by Serum Hexosaminidase Assay," *New England Journal of Medicine* 283 (2 July 1970): 15–20; John O'Brien, Shintaro Okada, Dorothy Fillerup, M. Lois Veath, Bruce Adornata, Paul Brenner, and Jules Leroy, "Tay-Sachs Disease: Prenatal Diagnosis," *Science* 172 (2 April 1971): 61–64.

29 N. C. Myrianthopoulos and S. M. Aronson, "Population Dynamics of Tay-Sachs Disease. I. Reproductive Fitness and Selection," *American Journal of Human Genetics* 18 (July 1966): 313–27; C. Sheba, "Jewish Migration in Its Historical Perspective," *Israel Journal of Medical Sciences* 7 (1971): 1333–41; Arlene Fraikor, "Tay-Sachs Disease: Genetic Drift among the Ashkenazim Jews," *Social Biology* 24 (1977): 117–34.

30 Fraikor, "Tay-Sachs Disease: Genetic Drift," 129, 131.

31 Jared Diamond, "Curse and Blessing of the Ghetto," *Discover*, March 1991, 60–65.

32 Diane Hamilton, "A Nursing Challenge: Adult-Onset Tay-Sachs Disease," *Archives of Psychiatric Nursing* 5 (December 1991): 382–85, at 382, quoting from an article by John S. O'Brien, "The Gangliosides," in *The Metabolic Basis of Inherited Disease*, ed. J. B. Stanburg (New York: McGraw Hill, 1983). See also P. L. Rosebush et al., "Late-Onset Tay-Sachs Disease Presenting as Catatonic Schizophrenia: Diagnostic and Treatment Issues," *Journal of Clinical Psychiatry* 56 (August 1995): 347–53. Distinct from the "classic infantile form of the disorder," patients with the "so-called juvenile form of the illness typically develop obvious signs and symptoms in early childhood (ages 1–9 years) and usually die in their midteens" (347). It also became clear that "other patients with hexosaminidase deficiency follow a less malignant clinical course and can live into adulthood" (347).

33 Friedman, "Tay-Sachs and Other Lipid Storage Diseases," 774.

34 J. F. Tallman, P. G. Pentcheve, and R. O. Brady, "An Enzymological Approach to the Lipidoses," *Enzyme* 18 (1974): 136–49; R. J. Desnick, R. W. Bernlohr, and W. Krivit, "Enzyme Therapy for Inborn Errors of Metabolism," *Postgraduate Medicine* 53 (1973): 214–16.

35 On ethical issues in Gaucher's testing, see, for example, Bowman, "Cultural and Ethnic Differences in Genetic Testing."

36 R. O. Brady, P. G. Pentcheve, and A. G. Gal, "Investigations in Enzyme Replacement Therapy in Lipid Storage Diseases," *Federation Proceedings* 34 (April 1975): 1310–15, at 1314. See also H. L. Nadler, "Current Status of Treatment in Storage Disorders," *Birth Defects: Original Articles Series* 12 (1976): 177–88, and P. G. Pentchev, "Enzyme Replacement Therapy in Gaucher's and Fabry's Disease," *Annals of Clinical and Laboratory Science* 7 (1977): 251–53.

37 J. M. Tager, M. N. Hamers, et al., "An Appraisal of Human Trials in Enzyme Therapy of Genetic Disease," *Birth Defects: Original Articles Series* 16 (1980): 343–59; R. O. Brady et al., "Status of Enzyme Replacement Therapy for Gaucher's Disease," *Birth Defects: Original Articles Series* 16 (1980): 361–68.

38 Robert J. Desnick and James Goldberg, "Tay-Sachs Disease: Prospects for Therapeutic Intervention," in *Tay-Sachs Disease*, ed. Kaback, 129–41, at 138.

39 E. Beutler and G. L. Dale, "Gaucher Disease: A Century of Delineation and Research. Enzyme Replacement Therapy: Model and Clinical Studies," *Progress in Clinical and Biological Research* 95 (1982): 703–16.

40 Desnick and Goldberg, "Tay-Sachs Disease," 137–38.

41 N. W. Barton et al., "Therapeutic Response to Intravenous Infusions of Glucocerebrosidase in a Patient with Gaucher Disease," *Proceedings of the National Academy of Sciences of the United States of America* 87 (1990): 1913–16; E. Beutler et al., "Enzyme Replacement Therapy for Gaucher Disease," *Blood* 78 (1991): 1183–89; A. C. Kay et al., "Enzyme Replacement Therapy in Type I Gaucher Disease," *Transactions of the Association of American Physicians* 104 (1991): 258–64.

42 J. M. Rappaport et al., "Bone Marrow Transplantation in Gaucher Disease," *Birth Defects: Original Article Series* 22 (1986): 101–9; P. V. Choudary et al., "The Molecular Biology of Gaucher Disease and the Potential for Gene Therapy," *Cold Spring Harbor Symposia on Quantitative Biology* 2 (1986): 2; O. C. Ringden et al., "Long-Term Follow-up of the First Successful Bone Marrow Transplantation in Gaucher Disease," *Transplantation* 46 (1988): 66–70; D. B. Kohn et al., "Toward Gene Therapy for Gaucher Disease," *Human Gene Therapy* 2 (1991): 101–5; O. C. Ringden et al., "Ten Years' Experience of Bone Marrow Transplantation for Gaucher Disease," *Transplantation* 59 (1995): 864–70; Ernest Beutler, "Newer Aspects of Some Interesting Lipid Storage Diseases: Tay-Sachs and Gaucher's Disease," *Western Journal of Medicine* 126 (January 1977):

53. "In the complex setting of far-advanced Gaucher's disease, the results of therapy are not easy to evaluate," noted Beutler. His article included no considerations of therapy in Tay-Sachs.

43 E. Beutler, "Economic Malpractice in the Treatment of Gaucher's Disease," *American Journal of Medicine* 97 (July 1994): 1–2.

44 Diane Paul, *Controlling Human Heredity, 1865 to the Present* (Atlantic Highlands, N.J.: Humanities Press, 1995).

45 See, for example, *An Act to Amend the Public Health Service Act to Provide for the Control of Sickle Cell Anemia* [National Sickle Cell Anemia Control Act], Public Law 92-294, 86 Stat. 138, 16 May 1972; *Cooley's Anemia Screening and Counseling Program: Hearing . . . to Amend the Public Health Service Act to Provide for the Prevention of Cooley's Anemia*, 92d Cong., 2d sess., 23 May 1972; *Hemophilia act of 1973: Hearing . . . to Amend the Public Health Service Act*, 93d Cong., 1st sess., 15 November 1973; *A Bill to Amend the Public Health Service Act to Provide for the Screening and Counseling of Americans with Respect to Tay-Sachs Disease*, H.R. 2569, 94th Cong., 1st sess., 3 February 1975; *A Bill to Amend the Public Health Service Act to Establish a National Program with Respect to Genetic Disease*, S. 1715, 94th Cong., 1st sess., 12 May 1975; *National Tay-Sachs Disease Screening and Counseling Act*, H.R. 2889, 96th Cong., 1st sess., 14 March 1979.

46 E. Beck, S. Blaichman, C. R. Scriver, and C. L. Clow, "Advocacy and Compliance in Genetic Screening," *New England Journal of Medicine* 291 (28 November 1974): 1166. See also Michael Kaback, "Heterozygote Screening: A Social Challenge," *New England Journal of Medicine* 289 (15 November 1973): 1090–91.

47 John O'Brien, "Tay-Sachs Disease: From Enzyme to Prevention," *Contributions of Neurochemistry to Neurology and Psychiatry* 32 (February 1973): 191–99.

48 James M. Gustafson, "Genetic Screening and Human Values: An Analysis," in *Ethical, Social, and Legal Dimensions of Screening for Human Genetic Disease*, ed. Daniel Bergsma (New York: Stratton Intercontinental Medical Book Corporation, 1974), 201–24, at 211.

49 Rabbi Roland B. Gittlesohn, president of the Central Conference of American (Reform) Rabbis, quoted in "Mixed Marriage Feelings," *Time*, 5 July 1971, 52. See also "Intermarriage Threatens American Jewish Community," *USA Today* 108, no. 2415 (December 1979): 10–11, and Marshall Sklare, "Intermarriage and Jewish Survival," *Commentary*, March 1970, 51–58.

50 G. Scheiderman, J. A. Lowden, and Q. Rae-Grant, "Tay-Sachs' and Related Lipid Storage Diseases: A Study of Families," *Canadian Psychiatric Association Journal* 18 (June 1973): 217.

51 "Poster Child Named," *New York Times*, 21 February 1972, sec. 2, p. 35; Frank Deford, *Alex: The Life of a Child* (New York: Viking, 1983).

52 Barbara Mahany, "Tay-Sachs Test Eases the Fears of Orthodox Jews," *Chicago Tribune*, 7 February 1994, 2.

53 William Curran, "Tay-Sachs Disease, Wrongful Life, and Preventive Malpractice," *American Journal of Public Health* 67 (June 1977): 568. As Curran notes, in one legal case in New York, a judge agreed with the parents of a TSD child that "the obstetrician did not take the proper steps to counsel them about the dangers they were running, or to conduct the necessary tests, or to perform or advise on an abortion."

54 Matthew Frye Jacobsen, *Whiteness of a Different Color: European Immigrants and the Alchemy of Race* (Cambridge, Mass.: Harvard University Press, 1998), 199; Brodkin, *How Jews Became White Folks*; Gilbert S. Rosenthal, *The Jewish Family in a Changing World* (New York: Thomas Yoseloff, 1970), quoted in Arlene Fraikor, "TSD and Life in New York City," in *Tay-Sachs Disease*, ed. Kaback, 119.

55 Desnick and Goldberg, "Tay-Sachs Disease," 138.

56 Frederick Hecht, "Screening People of Jewish Origin for Tay-Sachs Disease Carriers," *Arizona Medicine*, January 1981, 23–25.

57 R. M. Schmidt and W. J. Curran, "A National Genetic-Disease Program: Some Issues of Implementation," *New England Journal of Medicine* 293 (October 1976): 819–20.

58 Ibid., 820.

59 F. J. Ingelfinger, "Sounding Board: Cozening the People with Ambiguous Claims," *New England Journal of Medicine* 297 (August 1977): 334.

60 R. H. Kenen and R. M. Schmidt, "Stigmatization of Carrier Status: Social Implications of Heterozygote Genetic Screening Programs," *American Journal of Public Health* 68 (November 1978): 1119. The authors continued: "Two studies indicate that religious couples accept the birth of a child with a severe defect with fewer guilt feelings than do more secular oriented parents, the event being viewed as 'God's will'. Will these individuals be more likely to accept carrier status as God's will, thus alleviating their anxieties and feelings of inadequacy?"

61 Linus Pauling, "Reflections on a New Biology: Foreword," *UCLA Law Review* 15 (1968): 269. For more on this controversy, see Keith Wailoo,

Dying in the City of the Blues: Sickle Cell Anemia and the Politics of Race and Health (Chapel Hill: University of North Carolina Press, 2001), 186.

62 J. M. Swint, J. M. Shapiro, V. L. Corson, L. W. Reynolds, G. H. Thomas, and H. H. Kazazian, "The Economic Returns to Community and Hospital Screening Programs for Genetic Disease," *Preventive Medicine* 8 (1979): 463–70.

63 Madeleine Goodman and Lenn Goodman, "The Overselling of Genetic Anxiety," *Hastings Center Report*, October 1982, 20–27, at 20.

64 P. Carmody, M. Rattazzi, and R. Davidson, "Tay-Sachs Disease: The Use of Tears for the Detection of Heterozygotes," *New England Journal of Medicine* 289 (15 November 1973): 1072–74.

65 P. Steiner-Grossman and K. L. David, "Involvement of Rabbis in Counseling and Referral for Genetic Conditions: Results of a Survey," *American Journal of Human Genetics* 53 (1993): 1360.

66 Goodman and Goodman, "Overselling of Genetic Anxiety," 23.

67 Jane Feldman Paritzky, "Tay-Sachs: The Dreaded Inheritance," *American Journal of Nursing*, March 1985, 260–64.

68 E. D. Rosenstein, L. Godmilow, and K. Hirschhorn, "An Assessment of Physician Knowledge of Tay Sachs Disease," *Mount Sinai Journal of Medicine* 47 (January–February 1980): 1–4.

69 P. M. Tocci, "Seven Years Experience with Tay-Sachs Screening in Florida," *Journal of the Florida Medical Association* 68 (January 1981): 24–29.

70 Roscoe Brady, "Control and Therapy of Lipid Storage Diseases: Present Status and Future Strategies," *Alabama Journal of Medical Sciences* 19 (1982): 161–64.

71 B. Merz, "Matchmaking Scheme Solves Tay-Sachs Problem," *Journal of the American Medical Association* 258 (20 November 1987): 2636–37. As this article noted, "The rabbi proposed the idea to Robert Desnick . . . director of the Center for Jewish Genetic Diseases at Mount Sinai School of Medicine. Desnick was taken with the logic of the scheme and offered to assist in the organization of this novel screening program."

72 H. R. Spiers, "Community Consultation and AIDS Clinical Trials: I. IRB Rev.," *Human Subjects Research* 13, no. 3 (May–June 1991): 7–10; E. N. Dorff, "Jewish Theological and Moral Reflections on Genetic Screening: The Case of BRCA1," *Health Matrix* 7, no. 1 (winter 1997: 65–96.

73 Quoted in Judy Siegel-Itzkovich, "Genetic 'Matchmakers' Prevent

Tragedy," *Jerusalem Post*, 6 March 2003, 7. See also Kolata, "Using Genetic Tests, Ashkenazi Jews Vanquish a Disease."

74 E. Andermann, C. R. Scriver, L. S. Wolfe, L. Dansky, and F. Andermann, "Genetic Variants of Tay-Sachs Disease: Tay-Sachs Disease and Sandhoff's Disease in French Canadians, Juvenile Tay-Sachs Disease in Lebanese Canadians, and a Tay-Sachs Screening Program in the French-Canadian Population," in *Tay-Sachs Disease*, ed. Kaback, 161–88.

75 Quoted in George, "Rabbi's Dilemma," 44.

76 Steiner-Grossman and David, "Involvement of Rabbis in Counseling and Referral for Genetic Conditions."

77 The term *Ultra-Orthodox*, though controversial, often refers to Haredi Judaism or Hasidic Judaism—the most theologically conservative form of Judaism, whose adherents see themselves as linked in an unbroken chain back to Moses and the giving of the Torah on Mount Sinai. As a result, they often see non-Orthodox denominations as deviations from true Judaism and thus as not truly Jewish. On this tension, see Noah Efron and Norah Efron, *Real Jews: Secular versus Ultra-Orthodox: The Struggle for Jewish Identity in Israel* (New York: Basic Books, 2003). See also E. Broide, M. Zeigler, J. Ekstein, and G. Bach, "Screening for Carriers of Tay-Sachs Disease in the Ultraorthodox Ashkenazi Jewish Community in Israel," *American Journal of Medical Genetics* 47 (15 August 1993): 213–15.

78 Quoted in George, "Rabbi's Dilemma," 44.

79 Merz, "Matchmaking Scheme," 2639. See also J. Brown, "Prenatal Screening in Jewish Law," *Journal of Medical Ethics* 16 (1990): 75–80.

80 Gideon Back, chairman of the Human Genetics Hadasch University Hospital in Jerusalem and Dor Yeshorim board member, quoted in Netty Gross, "When the Genes Don't Match," *Jerusalem Report*, 7 March 2005, 20.

81 Mahany, "Tay-Sachs Test Eases Fears of Orthodox Jews," 1.

82 Siegel-Itzkovich, "Genetic 'Matchmakers' Prevent Tragedy," 7.

83 U.S. Congress, Office of Technology Assessment, *Cystic Fibrosis and DNA Tests*, 256.

84 Kolata, "Nightmare or the Dream of a New Era in Genetics?" A1.

85 Ibid. The reference to dating should not be understood as the common Western practice of two individuals meeting socially. In Orthodox communities it entails more carefully circumscribed meeting between the couple's parents or fathers.

86 Seigler and Collins both quoted in ibid.

87 Sura Jeselsohn, "In Genetics, Too, an Ounce of Prevention," letter to the editor, *New York Times*, 11 December 1993, A24.

88 See, for example, Robert J. Desnick, Mount Sinai School of Medicine, New York, "Genetic Testing in the Ashkenazi Jewish Population" (grant #R01 HG00644, grant period 4/1/93–3/31/96):

> The objective of this research is to conduct and evaluate a pilot program for the simultaneous screening of carriers for CF, TSD, and Gaucher's Disease in the Ashkenazi Jewish population. This ethnic group is unique since 95 percent of CF and GD carriers can be detected, providing the rationale to introduce CF and GD screening in conjunction with TSD carrier screening programs. This pilot study will address issues of education, improved and cost effective test methods, effective counseling and potential psychological harm, as well as ethical and health policy considerations. 10,000 Ashkenazi Jewish participants (about 5,000 couples) will be recruited for the study. Comparison of screening for these diseases will permit identification of screening issues related to differences in disease severity, availability of treatment, and detection accuracy for carrier couples.

89 Cornwell, "Jewish Marriage Makers Embrace Testing for Genetic Disease," 27.

90 Nicholas Wade, "Gene Mutation Tied to Colon Cancers in Ashkenazi Jews," *New York Times*, 26 August 1997, A1; Nicholas Wade, "Testing Genes to Save a Life without Costing You a Job," *New York Times*, 14 September 1997, WK5. The latter article explores "potential problems with discrimination arising from genetic testing . . . in light of recent discovery of test for genetic mutation that increases risk of colon cancer among Askenazi Jews."

91 Gina Kolata, "Bad Genes: A Cancer-Causing Mutation Is Found in European Jews," *New York Times*, 1 October 1995, sec. 4, p. 2; Richard Saltus, "Gene in Some Jewish Women Tied to Cancer Risk," *Boston Globe*, 29 September 1995, 1; Rick Weiss, "High Cancer Risk Found in Some Jewish Women," *Chicago Sun-Times*, 29 September 1995, 3. As one article noted, "Scientists have discovered a specific mutation in the BRCA-1 gene that apparently exists solely in Jews whose forebears came from eastern Europe, perhaps explaining why women in that

population are at elevated risk for breast cancer." "Ashkenazi Jewish Women Linked to Mutated Breast Cancer," *Buffalo News*, 30 August 1995, A6.

92 Quoted in Siegel-Itzkovich, "Genetic 'Matchmakers' Prevent Tragedies," 7.

93 Denise Grady, "Gene Identified as Major Cause of Deafness in Ashkenazi Jews," *New York Times*, 19 November 1998, A22.

94 Rabbi J. J. Rosner, quoted in Gross, "When the Genes Don't Match," 20.

95 D. Kronn et al., "Carrier Screening for Cystic Fibrosis, Gaucher Disease, and Tay-Sachs Disease in Askenazi Jewish Population: the First 1000 Cases at New York University Medical Center," *Archives of Internal Medicine* 158 (1998): 777–81.

96 Gross, "When the Genes Don't Match," 20.

97 S. Lehrman, "Jewish Leaders Seek Genetic Guidelines," *Nature* 389 (25 September 1997): 322; K. H. Rothenberg, "Breast Cancer, the Genetic Quick Fix, and the Jewish Community: Ethical, Legal, and Social Challenges," *Health Matrix* 7, no. 1 (winter 1997): 97–124.

98 Jim Ritter, "Genes May Be Leading Jews into Danger," *Chicago Sun-Times*, 28 November 1999, 10. On insurance and genetic discrimination, see, for example, Tina Hesman, "Genetic Tests Are Raising Privacy Issues: Discrimination by Insurance Firms, Employers Is Feared," *St. Louis Post-Dispatch*, 2 July 2000, A1.

99 Ritter, "Genes May Be Leading Jews into Danger," 10. Reports varied as to the actual number of diseases targeted by the Dor Yeshorim. A 2003 article in the *Jerusalem Post*, for example, mentions family dysautonomia, cystic fibrosis, Canavan's disease, Fanconi's anemia type C, glycogen storage disease, and Bloom's syndrome; Siegel-Itzkovich, "Genetic 'Matchmakers' Prevent Tragedies," 7. A 2000 article in the *St. Louis Post-Dispatch* mentions TSD, Canavan's disease, cystic fibrosis, and Fanconi's anemia; Hesman, "Genetic Tests Are Raising Privacy Issues," A1.

100 Tay-Sachs may be better known as a "Jewish genetic disease," but type I Gaucher's is in fact more prevalent among Ashkenazic Jews. Gaucher's is routinely said to be "the most common lipid storage disorder" as well as "the most common genetic disorder affecting Jewish people of Eastern European descent." National Gaucher Foundation website (http://www.gaucherdisease.org), accessed 11 July 2005. See

also Robert J. Desnick, "Gaucher Disease (1882–1982): Centennial Perspectives on the Most Prevalent Jewish Genetic Disease," *Mount Sinai Journal of Medicine* 49 (November–December 1982): 443–55.

101 N. C. Myrianthopoulos, "Molecular Approaches in the Prenatal Diagnosis and Therapy of Genetic Disorders," *Fetal Therapy* 2 (1987): 166; W. Krivit, C. B. Whitley, G. Lund, W. K. C. Ramsey, and J. H. Kersey, "Improvement of Clinical Expression of Central Nervous System Manifestations in Lysosomal Storage Diseases Treated by Bone Marrow Transplantation," in *Recent Advances and Future Directions in Bone Marrow Transplantation*, ed. S. J. Baum, G. W. Santos, and F. Takuku, (New York: Springer, 1987), 189–94. Gaucher's types II and III both have neurological involvement and are resistant to treatment by enzyme replacement. Insofar as there was hope at all in the 1980s for enzyme replacement treatment for lysosomal storage disorders, it was in Gaucher's type I.

102 The disease was discovered by a French medical student named Philippe Charles Ernest Gaucher. Upon postmortem examination of a patient, Gaucher found that the cells in the spleen were swollen. Those enlarged cells (now called Gaucher cells) became the telltale sign of the disease. Gaucher described his clinical and pathological findings in his doctoral thesis, allowing other physicians to diagnose the condition.

103 Robert Reingold, "Drugs That Promise Help but Not Profit Reside in Limbo," *New York Times*, 17 March 1981, C1.

104 M. L. Figueroa et al., "A Less Costly Regimen of Alglucerase to Treat Gaucher's Disease," *New England Journal of Medicine* 327 (1992): 1632–36; A. M. Garber, "No Price Too High?" *New England Journal of Medicine* 327 (1992): 1676–78; A. Zimran et al., "Home Treatment with Intravenous Enzyme Replacement Therapy for Gaucher Disease: An International Collaborative Study of 33 Patients," *Blood* 82 (1993): 1107–9.

105 Kolata, "Nightmare or the Dream of a New Era in Genetics?" A1.

106 D. P. Goldman, A. E. Clarke, and A. M. Garber, "Creating the Costliest Orphan: The Orphan Drug Act in the Development of Ceredase," *International Journal of Technology Assessment in Health Care* 8 (1992): 583–97.

107 A chronology of the story of Genzyme and Ceredase can be found in Ronald Rosenberg, "Biotechnology: Genzyme to Raise Profile, Stakes Company Facing Growth Challenges," *Boston Globe*, 20 September 2000, E4.

108 Ibid.

109 Ekstein quoted in Kolata, "Nightmare or the Dream of a New Era in Genetics?" A1.

110 The attitude toward Gaucher's in Israel is perhaps the best example of a nation taking communal responsibility for a disease. Gaucher's is one of four serious diseases covered by Israeli national health insurance. Care for the disease is very expensive, akin to that for hemophilia, kidney disease, and thalassemia. A report in the *Jerusalem Post* on genetic disease testing and prevention that did not include Gaucher's elicited a revealing response from an American concerned about this omission. Writing from the Yale University Gaucher's Disease Center, Wayne Rosenfield inquired of the author, "You omitted any mention of Gaucher Disease . . . the most common genetic disorder among the Jewish people, with a carrier rate of 1 in 14 Jews of Eastern European ancestry." The author replied that testing for Gaucher's was not the norm in Israel and did not fall under the testing practices of the Dor Yeshorim: "The organization does not test for Gaucher's, as this is not considered a reason for not marrying. Today's treatments for Gaucher's, which in Israel are covered by the basket of health services provided by the public health funds, are very effective." Screening for Gaucher's would merely cause "needless anxiety." Siegel-Itzkovich, "Genetic 'Matchmakers' Prevent Tragedies," 7.

111 Ekstein quoted in George, "Rabbi's Dilemma," 44. Commenting on the patenting of genes and the profit motive in genetic disease testing and management, Ekstein noted that "companies sometimes get greedy and charge way too much, which can prevent people from taking a test."

112 Quoted in Kolata, "Bad Genes," 2.

113 See, for example, Tarek Hamada, "Thousands of Jews Use Genetics to Track an Elusive Deadly Killer," *Detroit News*, 17 December 1993, B1.

114 Consider, for example, the writing of Jared Diamond. Other authors have characterized the spectrum of "Jewish genetic diseases" as having conferred similar benefits. While such theories are built on historical associations and grand speculation, they nonetheless exemplify the continuing impulse to use genetics to link people's imagined past to their vital present. Diamond, "Curse and Blessing of the Ghetto"; Josie Glausiusz, "Unfortunate Drift," *Discover*, June 1995, 34–35. See also Rick Weiss, "Discovery of 'Jewish' Cancer Gene Raises Fears of More Than Disease," *Washington Post*, 3 September 1997, A1; Karen Rafin-

ski, "Early Warning," *Chicago Tribune*, 5 June 1997, 2; and Gina Kolata, "Breast Cancer Gene in 1% of U.S. Jews," *New York Times*, 29 September 1995, A24; Nicholas Wade, "Researchers Say Intelligence and Diseases May Be Linked in Ashkenazic Genes," *New York Times*, 3 June 2005, A21.

115 Arthur Beaudet, "Gaucher's Disease," *New England Journal of Medicine* 316 (5 March 1987): 620.

116 "Healthy Baby Is Born after Test for Deadly Gene," *New York Times*, 28 January 1994, A17.

CHAPTER 2. RISKY BUSINESS IN WHITE AMERICA

1 Natalie Angier, "Gene Therapy Begins for Fatal Lung Disease: Cystic Fibrosis Patient Inhales Altered Cold Virus," *New York Times*, 20 April 1993, C5.

2 Quoted in Gina Kolata, "Nightmare or the Dream of a New Era in Genetics?" *New York Times*, 7 December 1993, A1.

3 Such descriptions could be found in medical articles, scientific treatises, and popular media. For example, one author wrote, "CF is most prevalent among people of Central European ancestry . . . and is somewhat less common in Scandinavia." Yet the author also noted that CF had been reported in about 1 in 17,000 black Americans, and 1 in 90,000 Asians (mainly Japanese) in Hawaii, but that the prevalence of CF in Asia and Africa had not been adequately investigated: "It is possible that its true prevalence is masked by high infant mortality in large populations of these continents." Thomas G. Benedek, "Cystic Fibrosis," in *The Cambridge Historical Dictionary of Disease*, ed. Kenneth F. Kiple (New York: Cambridge University Press, 2003), 84. See also Tim Beardsley, "Clearing the Airways: Cystic Fibrosis May Be Treated with Gene Therapy," *Scientific American*, December 1990, 28 ("most common genetic disease of white people"); Purvis, "Laying Siege to a Deadly Gene," 60 ("most common inherited disorder among whites"); and Jeannette Dankert-Roelse and Gerard Te Meerman, "Screening for Cystic Fibrosis: Time to Change Our Position?" *New England Journal of Medicine* 337 (2 October 1997): 997 ("one of the most common inheritable diseases among white people").

4 B. Kerem, J. M. Rommens, J. A. Buchanan, D. Markiewicz, T. K. Cox, A. Chakravarti, M. Buchwald, and L. C. Tsui, "Identification of the Cystic Fibrosis Gene: Genetic Analysis," *Science* 245 (8 September 1989): 1073–80. Thus, one should speak not of a CF gene but of a wide range

of genetic mutations resulting in the diverse phenomena known as cystic fibrosis. Xavier Estivill, Consul Bancells, Cristina Ramos, and the Biomed CF Mutation Analysis Consortium, "Geographic Distribution and Regional Origin of 272 Cystic Fibrosis Mutations in European Populations," *Human Mutation* 10 (1997): 135–54, at 152. In such studies the tendency has been to focus not on the distribution of CF itself but on that percentage of CF patients carrying the DF508 gene—a distinct subset of the larger CF population.

5 Genoveva Keyeux et al., "CFTR Mutations in Patients from Colombia: Implications for Local and Regional Molecular Diagnosis Programs," *Human Mutation* 22 (September 2003): 259. As another study from Latin America concluded, "Our data suggest that CF mutations in Ecuador . . . have a different ethiology [sic] from that of Caucasian populations. This may be the consequence of a different genetic background in Latin America . . . [where] the most important ethnic groups are 'mestizo' [mixture of Spaniard and Amerindian] and Amerindian." Cesar Paz-y-Mino et al., "The Delta F508 Mutation in Ecuador, South America," *Human Mutation* 14 (1999): 348.

6 Estivill et al., "Geographic Distribution and Regional Origin," 147.

7 One 1992 study, for example, turned attention to the Basque population, one of the oldest ethnic subgroups in Europe, noting that "the frequency of the DF 508 mutation in the chromosomes of Basque origin is 87%, compared with 58% in those of Mixed Basque origin." This exceptionally high percentage of the gene among CF patients suggested that the mutation itself was of ancient European pedigree, "already present in Europe more than 10,000 years ago." T. Casals et al., "Cystic Fibrosis in the Basque Country: High Frequency of Mutation DF508 in Patients of Basque Origin" *American Journal of Human Genetics* 50 (1992): 404–10, at 404. Another 1992 study used the gene's frequency as a basis for scrutinizing the Irish population, bringing a layer of supposed genetic understanding to Ireland's political and religious divisions. The study concluded that "although the populations of the Republic of Ireland (mostly of Protestant faith) and of Northern Ireland (mostly of Catholic faith) had the same CF incidence (1 in 1800), they differed in the proportion of the DF508 mutation (75% and 54% respectively)." The implications of such findings remained unclear; some might infer that the Irish Protestants were more European than the Irish Catholics of Northern Ireland. Marc De Braekeleer

and Jocelyne Daignealt, "Spacial Distribution of the DF508 Mutation in Cystic Fibrosis: A Review," *Human Biology*, 64 (2 April 1992): 169–70.

8 Robert Schulman et al., "The Gene Doctors: Scientists Are on the Verge of Curing Life's Cruelest Diseases," *Business Week*, 18 November 1985, 76–80; Natalie Angier, "Panel Permits Use of Genes in Treating Cystic Fibrosis," *New York Times*, 4 December 1992, A28; Angier, "Gene Therapy Begins for Fatal Lung Disease"; Geoffrey Cowley, "Closing in on Cystic Fibrosis: Researchers Are Learning to Replace a Faulty Gene," *Newsweek*, 3 May 1993, 56.

9 Elyse Tanouye, "Majority Supports Gene-Based Therapy, New Survey Shows," *Wall Street Journal*, 29 September 1992, B10. This article reports on a survey sponsored by the March of Dimes Birth Defects Foundation, which found that 89 percent of Americans supported the use of gene therapy to treat disease. More than 40 percent approved of using gene therapy to enhance the physical and mental characteristics of healthy people. A majority also felt that genetic test results need not be confidential and that employers and insurance companies had a right to know them. The article noted that Americans approve of gene-based research and therapy even though "many don't understand much about science." Dr. Howse of the March of Dimes Birth Defects Foundation is quoted in the article as saying, "The foundation believes that gene therapy represents a fundamental leap forward in the cure and treatment of birth defects."

10 Joe Palca, "The Promise of a Cure," *Discover*, June 1994, 75–86.

11 Mark Nichols, "A Test Case in Hope: A New Treatment Could Cure Cystic Fibrosis," *Maclean's*, 3 May 1993, 39.

12 Leon Jaroff and Hannah Bloch, "Keys to the Kingdom," *Time* 148, no. 14, *Fall 1996 Special Issue*, 24–29; Anderson quoted at 28. Francis Collins has also endorsed this perspective. In Jean Seligmann, "Curing Cystic Fibrosis? Genes Convert Sick Cells," *Newsweek*, 1 October 1990, 64, he is quoted as saying that "the new CF research shows that the [gene therapy] strategy works for an ever-increasing list of disorders where a defective gene is responsible . . . It gives credence to the idea that gene therapy will find a significant place in the therapeutic armamentarium."

13 "'I don't think chloride regulation is the sole defect, and I'm not sure it's the primary pathology,' cautioned Richard C. Boucher . . . Boucher pointed out that CF patients fall prey to characteristic infections

not found in patients with other lung diseases. To him, that suggested there may be more to CF than a failure to clear lung mucus." Tim Beardsley, "Clearing the Airways: Cystic Fibrosis May Be Treated with Gene Therapy," *Scientific American*, December 1990, 29–30. Gene therapy for CF involves delivery of a cystic fibrosis transmembrane regulator (CFTR) gene to the membrane of cells lining the airways of the lungs. It was suspected that the inability of CF patients to regulate chloride ions leads to the lung mucus characteristic of this disease. Sodium ion regulation is also impaired in the CF patient.

14 Quoted in Andrew Purvis, "Laying Siege to a Deadly Gene: Thanks to Series of Breakthroughs, Doctors Are Closing in on a Cure for Cystic Fibrosis," *Time*, 24 February 1992, 60–61.

15 Nancy King, Larry Churchill, Myra Collins, Keith Wailoo, and Stephen Pemberton, "Genetic Research as Therapy: Implications of 'Gene Therapy' for Informed Consent," *Journal of Law, Medicine, and Ethics* 26 (spring 1998): 38–47.

16 Ellen Lee, "On the Front Lines against Cystic Fibrosis," *Atlanta Journal and Constitution*, 23 August 1998, 4C.

17 Michael Kernan, "A Death in the Family: Frank Deford's Poignant Goodbye to His Daughter," *Washington Post*, 27 October 1983, D1.

18 Frank Deford, *Alex: The Life of a Child* (New York: Viking, 1983), 32.

19 Ibid., 43.

20 A useful overview of the therapeutic history of CF can be found in Carl Doershuk, ed., *Cystic Fibrosis in the Twentieth Century: People, Events, and Progress* (Cleveland, Ohio: AM Publishing, 2001). The framing of disease has a specific place in the recent history and historiography of medicine. See, for example, Charles E. Rosenberg, "Framing Disease: Illness, Society, and History," introduction to *Framing Disease: Studies in Cultural History*, ed. Charles E. Rosenberg and Janet Golden (New Brunswick: Rutgers University Press, 1992), xiii–xxvi.

21 Paul A. di Sant' Agnese, "Experiences of a Pioneer Researcher: Discovery of the Sweat Electrolyte Defect and the Early Medical History of Cystic Fibrosis," in *Cystic Fibrosis in the Twentieth Century*, ed. Doershuk, 17–35, at 18. Historical accounts of the disease do occasionally claim that people recognized CF in some form before the 1930s — particularly in the form of salty sweat. Thomas Benedek recently claimed that CF was probably recognized many centuries ago, for "according to a medi-

eval German saying, 'The infant who when kissed leaves a taste of salt will not reach the first year of life.'" Benedek, "Cystic Fibrosis," 84.

22 Dorothy H. Anderson, "Cystic Fibrosis of the Pancreas and Its Relation to Celiac Disease: A Clinical and Pathological Study," *American Journal of the Diseases of Children* 56 (1938): 344–99. The standard treatment for CF in the 1940s and 1950s was a "low fat and high protein diet, vitamins, pancreatin to replace the missing pancreatic enzymes, and tetracycline for antibiotic therapy." Carl F. Doershuk, "The Matthews Comprehensive Treatment Program: A Ray of Hope," in *Cystic Fibrosis in the Twentieth Century*, ed. Doershuk, 70.

23 Sidney Farber, "Some Organic Digestive Disturbances in Early Life," *Journal of the Michigan Medical Society* 44 (1945): 587–94. See also Sidney Farber, "Pancreatic Function and Disease in Early Life. V. Pathologic Changes Associated with Pancreatic Insufficiency in Early Life," *Archives of Pathology* 37 (1944): 238–50. Farber performed eighty-seven autopsies on infants and children with pancreatic insufficiencies. He noted pathologic changes in the lungs, upper respiratory tract, liver, gallbladder, and upper alimentary tract that were similar to those in the pancreas. He concluded, at the time, that CF was a systemic disease with a variety of clinical appearances. The clinical manifestations of CF changed relative to what organs were affected by mucolytic obstructions.

24 In the electrolyte test, Paul di Sant' Agnese and his associates provided a diagnostic standard for quantifying the abnormal salt loss found in the perspiration of some CF patients. See di Sant' Agnese, "Experiences of a Pioneer Researcher"; also P. di Sant' Agnese, R. Darling, G. Perera, et al., "Abnormal Electrolyte Composition of Sweat in Cystic Fibrosis of the Pancreas," *Pediatrics* 12 (1953): 549–63.

25 Kenneth S. Landauer, foreword to *Guide to Diagnosis and Management of Cystic Fibrosis: A Syllabus for Physicians* (New York: National Cystic Fibrosis Research Foundation, 1963), vi.

26 "'New' Disease," *Time*, 1 March 1954, quoted in Doershuk, "Matthews Comprehensive Treatment Program," 70–71. On the early history of CF, see also D. A. Christie and E. M. Tansey, eds., *Cystic Fibrosis: Wellcome Witnesses to Twentieth Century Medicine, Volume 20* (London: Wellcome Trust Centre for the History of Medicine at University College, London, 2004).

27 Paul A. di Sant' Agnese, "Cystic Fibrosis: The Problem and the Challenge," in Paul A. di Sant' Agnese, ed., *Research on Pathogenesis of Cystic Fibrosis of the Pancreas (Mucoviscidosis): Proceedings of the Third International Conference on Cystic Fibrosis*, Bethesda, Md., 28–30 September 1964, xxiii.

28 Landauer, foreword to *Guide to Diagnosis and Management of Cystic Fibrosis*, vi.

29 Doershuk, "Matthews Comprehensive Treatment Program," 63–78.

30 David J. Rothman, *Strangers at the Bedside: A History of How Law and Bioethics Transformed Medical Decision Making* (New York: Basic Books, 1991), 141.

31 Doershuk, "Matthews Comprehensive Treatment Program," 73.

32 *Guide to Diagnosis and Management of Cystic Fibrosis*.

33 Maarten S. Sibinga, C. Jack Friedman, and Nancy N. Huang, "The Family of the Cystic Fibrosis Patient," in *Psychosocial Aspects of Cystic Fibrosis: A Model for Chronic Lung Disease*, ed. Paul R. Patterson, Carolyn R. Denning, and Austin H. Kutscher (New York: Columbia University Press, 1973), 13–18.

34 Cynthia Mikkelsen, Eugenia Waechter, and Mary Crittenden, "Cystic Fibrosis: A Family Challenge," *Children Today*, July–August 1978, 22–26. The literature on CF was circumscribed by a range of parent-centered questions, from the challenges of home diagnosis and home management, to the topic of family communication about CF, to the difficult issue of sibling reactions to CF, and to CF children's relationship with peers, their understanding of hospitalization, and their sources of emotional support.

35 Atul Gawande, "The Bell Curve," *New Yorker*, 6 December 2004, 82–91.

36 Gus Cezeaux Jr., Jane Telford, Gunyon Harrison, and Arthur S. Keats, "Bronchial Lavage in Cystic Fibrosis: A Comparison of Agents," *Journal of the American Medical Association* 199 (2 January 1967): 73–76.

37 J. Lieberman, "Dornase Aerosol Effect on Sputum Viscosity in Cases of Cystic Fibrosis," *Journal of the American Medical Association* 205 (1968): 312–13.

38 See Paul di Sant' Agnese, "Guest Editorial: Fertility and the Young Adult with Cystic Fibrosis," *New England Journal of Medicine* 279 (1968): 103–5, and Elvin Kaplan et al., "Reproductive Failures in Males with Cystic Fibrosis," *New England Journal of Medicine* 279 (1968): 65–69.

39 Audrey T. McCollum and Lewis E. Gibson, "Family Adaptation to the

Child with Cystic Fibrosis," *Journal of Pediatrics* 77 (October 1970): 571–78. See also Hilaire J. Meuwissen, letter to the editor, *Journal of Pediatrics* 78 (March 1971): 548–49.

40 Deford, *Alex*, 37.

41 Mikkelsen, Waechter, and Crittenden, "Cystic Fibrosis: A Family Challenge."

42 Rustin McIntosh, ed., *Research on Cystic Fibrosis: Transactions of the International Research Conference on Cystic Fibrosis*, Washington, D.C., 7–9 January 1959 (Baltimore, Md.: French-Bray, 1960), xii.

43 Di Sant' Agnese, "Cystic Fibrosis: The Problem and the Challenge," xxiii–xxiv.

44 "Excerpt: Testimony of Dr. Merlin K. DuVal," in *National Heart, Blood Vessel, Lung, and Blood Act of 1972: Hearings before the Subcommittee on Public Health and Environment of the Committee on Interstate and Foreign Commerce, House of Representatives, 92nd U.S. Congress, H.R. 12571, 13715, 12460, 13500, S. 3323 (and Identical Bills) to Amend the Public Health Service Act . . . April 25–26, 1972*, serial no. 92-71 (Washington, D.C.: U.S. Government Printing Office, 1972), 89.

45 Ibid., 90.

46 Dr. Robert Scott, quoted in Nancy Hicks, "Doctor Asks Curb of Negro Disease," *New York Times*, 27 October 1970, A51.

47 "Statement of Giulio J. Barbero, M.D., Chairman, Department of Pediatrics, Hahnemann Medical College, Philadelphia, PA," in *National Heart, Blood Vessel, Lung, and Blood Act of 1972*, 216.

48 Ibid., 217.

49 For more details on this tension, see "Statement of Giulio J. Barbero" and "Excerpt: Testimony of Dr. Merlin K. DuVal," 89.

50 "Poster Child Named," *New York Times*, 21 February 1972, sec. 2, p. 35.

51 The legislation was a powerful symbolic statement of concern for pain and suffering in black America. See Keith Wailoo, *Dying in the City of the Blues: Sickle Cell Anemia and the Politics of Race and Health* (Chapel Hill: University of North Carolina Press, 2001).

52 "Statement of Giulio J. Barbero," 218–19.

53 To be sure, there were exceptions. Researchers in Minnesota continued to explore its prevalence among Scandinavian Americans, people of Northern European descent, and other Europeans. See *Chronic Respiratory Diseases in Children and Adolescents*, special issue of *Minnesota Medicine* 52 (September 1969).

54 See Robert C. Stern et al., "Course of Cystic Fibrosis in Black Patients," *Journal of Pediatrics* 89 (September 1976): 412–17; Ernest T. Heffer, "Cystic Fibrosis in Black Children," letter to the editor, *Journal of Pediatrics* 90 (February 1977); Lucas L. Kulczycki, "Incidence of Cystic Fibrosis in Black Children — Revisited," letter to the editor, *Journal of Pediatrics* 92 (May 1978): 855; and Clifford W. Lober, Hilliard F. Seigler, and Alexander Spock, "Cystic Fibrosis in a Black Woman," *Journal of the American Medical Association* 235 (15 March 1976): 1140–41.

55 Sterling Garrard, Julius Richmond, and Marvin Hirsch, "*Pseudomonas aeruginosa* Infection as a Complication of Therapy in Pancreatic Fibrosis (Mucoviscidosis)," *Pediatrics*, October 1951, 485.

56 M. W. Burns and J. R. May, "Bacterial Precipitin in Serum of Patients with Cystic Fibrosis, *Lancet*, 1968, no. 1:270–72.

57 Deford, *Alex*, 41.

58 Lucas Kulczycki, Thomas Murphy, and Joseph Bellanti, "*Pseudomonas* Colonization in Cystic Fibrosis: A Study of 160 Patients," *Journal of the American Medical Association* 240 (1978): 30–34.

59 Bernard Boxerbaum, Carl Doershuk, and LeRoy Matthews, "Use of Antibictics [sic] in Cystic Fibrosis," letter to the editor, *Journal of Pediatrics* 81 (July 1972): 188.

60 Editor's commentary on Pierre Beaudry, Melvin Marks, Dianne McDougall, et al., "Is Anti-*Pseudomonas* Therapy Warranted in Acute Respiratory Exacerbations in Children with Cystic Fibrosis?" *Journal of Pediatrics* 97 (July 1980): 148; text of article at 144–47.

61 Warren J. Warwick, "Cystic Fibrosis: An Expanding Challenge for Internal Medicine," *Journal of the American Medical Association* 238 (14 November 1977): 2159–62.

62 Kulczycki, Murphy, and Bellanti, "*Pseudomonas* Colonization in Cystic Fibrosis," 34.

63 Michael Parry, Harold Neu, Mario Melino, et al., "Treatment of Pulmonary Infections in Patients with Cystic Fibrosis: A Comparative Study of Ticarcillin and Gentamicin," *Journal of Pediatrics* 90 (January 1977): 144–48.

64 Vera A. Loening-Baucke, Elaine Mischler, and Martin G. Myers, "A Placebo-Controlled Trial of Cephalexin Therapy in the Ambulatory Management of Patients with Cystic Fibrosis," *Journal of Pediatrics* 95 (October 1979): 630–37.

65 Alexander Hyatt, Bradley Chipps, Karen Kumor, et al., "A Double-Blind

Controlled Trial of Anti-*Pseudomonas* Chemotherapy of Acute Respiratory Exacerbations in Patients with Cystic Fibrosis," *Journal of Pediatrics* 99 (August 1981): 307–11.

66 See Gregory L. Kearns et al., "Dosing Implications of Altered Gentamicin Disposition in Patients with Cystic Fibrosis," *Journal of Pediatrics* 100 (February 1982): 312–18, and G. Nolan et al., "Antibiotic Prophylaxis in Cystic Fibrosis: Inhaled Cephaloridine as an Adjunct to Oral Cloxacillin," *Journal of Pediatrics* 101 (October 1982): 626–30.

67 Rita Padoan et al., "Cefatrizine in Treatment of Acute Pulmonary Exacerbations in Patients with Cystic Fibrosis," *Journal of Pediatrics* 103 (August 1983): 320.

68 Richard B. Moss et al., "Allergy to Semisynthetic Penicillins in Cystic Fibrosis," *Journal of Pediatrics* 104 (March 1984): 460–66.

69 A. Isles et al., "*Pseudomonas cepacia* Infection in Cystic Fibrosis: An Emerging Problem," *Journal of Pediatrics* 104 (February 1984): 206–10.

70 R. Wientzen, C. Prestidge, R. I. Kramer, G. H. McCracken, and J. D. Nelson, "Acute Pulmonary Exacerbations in Cystic Fibrosis: A Double-Blind Trial of Tobramycin and Placebo Therapy," *American Journal of the Diseases of Children* 134 (1980): 1134.

71 John D. Nelson, discussion to "Management of Acute Pulmonary Exacerbations in Cystic Fibrosis: A Critical Appraisal," *Journal of Pediatrics* 106 (June 1985): 1033–34; text of article at 1030–33.

72 Kevin Gaskin et al., "Improved Respiratory Prognosis in Patients with Cystic Fibrosis with Normal Fat Absorption," *Journal of Pediatrics* 100 (June 1982): 857–62. See also Giulio Barbero's accompanying commentary on 914–15.

73 Anthony K. Webb, "Management Problems of the Adult with Cystic Fibrosis," *Journal Suisse de Médicine* 121 (1991): 110.

74 W. H. Frist et al., "Cystic Fibrosis Treated with Heart-Lung Transplantation: North American Results," *Transplantation Proceedings* 23 (February 1991): 1205–6.

75 On the impact of cyclosporine, see Renee Fox and Judith Swazey, *Spare Parts: Organ Replacement in American Society* (New York: Oxford University Press, 1992). See also R. Y. Calne, D. J. White, S. Thiru, et al., "Cyclosporin A in Patients Receiving Renal Allografts from Cadaveric Donors," *Lancet*, 1978, no. 2:1323–27.

76 Robert M. Kotloff and Jonathan B. Zuckerman, "Lung Transplantation for Cystic Fibrosis: Special Considerations," *Chest* 109 (March 1996):

787–88. See also Stanley Fiel et al., "Heart-Lung Transplantation in Cystic Fibrosis: Overview," *Clinical Transplants* 3 (1989): 162–63.

77 "Insurers Debating Transplant Costs: As Success of Surgery Rises, Medicare and Private Plan Payment Is Restudied," *New York Times*, 21 November 1983, A20.

78 Lindsey Gurson, "Center for Transplants Aids Pittsburgh Ascent," *New York Times*, 16 September 1985, A10. Gurson writes, "Many large teaching hospitals perceive [transplants] as vital to retaining preeminence." See also Tessa Melvin, "Surgeon Stresses Role of Donors," *New York Times*, 30 November 1986, Westchester Weekly section, 641–42; "Lag Seen in Transplants," *New York Times*, 5 November 1991, C7; and Barbara Stewart, "Hospitals Press for Expansion of Organ Transplant Units," *New York Times*, 24 November 1996, NJ6.

79 See, for example, Perri Klass, "Shattered Dreams," *Discover*, July 1988, 34–35. Klass, an adolescent medicine specialist, discussed the centrality of antibiotics not only in clinical management but in the changing power relations between CF adolescents and their caregivers. "Kids with cystic fibrosis come into the hospital fairly regularly, whenever their lungs start getting worse," she wrote. "They get what we call a cleanout, a course of multiple, very strong antibiotics, aimed at eradicating the particularly vicious organisms that grow in their lungs." Klass noted that the administration of intravenous antibiotics, however, was complicated by the desire of CF adolescents for control over the terms of therapy: "By the time these kids reach their teens, they know a hell of a lot about IVs . . . They pick a resident whose skills they approve of. They specify how many times they'll allow the resident to try inserting the new IV before they'll demand to see a senior resident. Finally they indicate precisely which vein on which arm is available for the next IV." Klass's observations highlight the continued complexity of managing CF, even in the clinical context, as patients became older and more independent.

80 Stanley B. Fiel, "Heart-Lung Transplantation for Patients with Cystic Fibrosis: A Test of Clinical Wisdom," *Archives of Internal Medicine* 151 (May 1991): 870.

81 Claudia Wells and Dick Thompson, "Hearts of the Matter," *Time*, 25 May 1987, 60. The advent of lung transplantation in cystic fibrosis had certainly captured public attention. News accounts followed the stories of patients who took this daring chance at survival. In some

cases the stories revealed the willingness of families to offer their own organs in order to postpone the death of their children. In other cases, lung transplantation operations even sought to address the lung deterioration preemptively, well before damage had set in. Some surgical specialists branched out to liver transplants, a possible consideration for a tiny minority of CF patients.

82 An article in *Redbook*, the magazine for parents, reported on two divorced parents who decided to reconcile in order to donate lungs because they "were the best biological matches." Noted one parent, "We gave him life once, and we can do it again." Sally Stich, "No Time for Regrets," *Redbook*, April 1994, 188.

83 William Plummer and Giovanna Breu, "A New Breath of Life," *People*, 6 July 1992, 118.

84 Quoted in ibid.

85 Frist et al., "Cystic Fibrosis Treated with Heart-Lung Transplantation."

86 Fiel, "Heart-Lung Transplantation for Patients with Cystic Fibrosis," 872.

87 Quoted in Plummer and Breu, "New Breath of Life," 118.

88 D. E. Koshland, "The Cystic Fibrosis Gene Story," *Science* 245 (8 September 1989): 1029; Kerem et al., "Identification of the Cystic Fibrosis Gene: Genetic Analysis"; J. M. Rommens, M. C. Iannuzzi, B. Kerem, M. L. Drumm, G. Melmer, M. Dean, R. Rozmahel, J. L. Cole, D. Kennedy, N. Hidaka, M. Zsiga, M. Buchwald, J. R. Riordan, L. C. Tsui, and F. S. Collins, "Identification of the Cystic Fibrosis Gene: Chromosome Walking and Jumping," *Science* 245 (8 September 1989): 1059–65; Jean Seligmann and Daniel Glick, "Cystic Fibrosis: Hunting Down a Killer Gene," *Newsweek*, 4 September 1989, 60–61.

89 Shulman et al., "Gene Doctors." See also Pat Ohlendorf, "The Taming of a Once-Certain Killer," *Maclean's* 98 (7 October 1985): 50, 52.

90 Harold Schmeck, "Genetic Marker for Cystic Fibrosis Reported Found," *New York Times*, 11 October 1995, A17.

91 Ibid.

92 Gene therapy also blurred the line between experiment and therapy. See Larry Churchill, Myra Collins, Nancy King, Stephen Pemberton, and Keith Wailoo, "Genetic Research as Therapy: Implications of 'Gene Therapy' for Informed Consent," *Journal of Law, Medicine, and Ethics* 26 (spring 1998): 38–47; and Nancy King, "Experimental Treatment: Oxymoron or Aspiration?" *Hastings Center Report* 25 (1995): 6–15.

93 Gina Kolata, "Progress Is Cited on Cystic Fibrosis," *New York Times,* 15 October 1993, A24.

94 Diane Brady, "Signals of Hope: Gene Therapy May Cure Cystic Fibrosis," *Maclean's,* 1 October 1990, 52; Jean Seligmann, "Curing Cystic Fibrosis? Genes Convert Sick Cells," *Newsweek,* 1 October 1990, 64; Mark Nichols, "A Test Case in Hope," *Maclean's,* 3 May 1993, 39. As one *Wall Street Journal* reporter noted in 1992, "The vast majority of Americans support the use of gene-based therapy to treat disease, even though they don't know much about the emerging science, according to a new survey." Elyse Tanouye, "Majority Supports Gene-Based Therapy," *Wall Street Journal,* 29 September 1992, B10.

95 Angier, "Gene Therapy Begins for Fatal Lung Disease," C5. See also Angier, "Panel Permits Use of Genes."

96 Geoffrey Cowley, "Closing in on Cystic Fibrosis: Researchers Are Learning to Replace a Faulty Gene," *Newsweek,* 3 May 1993, 56.

97 W. French Anderson stated in 1996, "Twenty years from now, gene therapy will have revolutionized the practice of medicine . . . Virtually every disease will have gene therapy as one of its treatments." Quoted in Jaroff and Bloch, "Keys to the Kingdom," 28.

98 Quotations all from Purvis, "Laying Siege to a Deadly Gene," 60–61.

99 Joan O'C. Hamilton, "A Star Drug Is Born," *Business Week,* 23 August 1993, 66–68.

100 "F.D.A. Approval Sought for Cystic Fibrosis Drug," *New York Times,* 31 March 1993, D4. See also "Drug by Genentech Gets Orphan Status," *New York Times,* 30 January 1991, D4.

101 John Carey, "The $600 Million Horse Race," *Business Week,* 23 August 1993, 68.

102 Natalie Angier, "Cystic Fibrosis: Experiment Hits a Snag," *New York Times,* 22 September 1993, C12. "To think we're going to cure cystic fibrosis in a year is naïve," Dr. Crystal was quoted as saying. "I'm not discouraged but this is going to take time and people shouldn't have unrealistic expectations."

103 Palca, "Promise of a Cure," 86.

104 Eliot Marshall, "Gene Therapy's Growing Pains: The Trouble with Vectors," *Science* 269 (25 August 1995): 1050–54, at 1052.

105 Palca, "Promise of a Cure."

106 Ibid.

107 Marshall, "Gene Therapy's Growing Pains."

108 Palca, "Promise of a Cure," 76. This phrase is the subtitle of Palca's essay.

109 Marshal, "Gene Therapy's Growing Pains," 1055.

110 Leo Furcht, "Industry: A Vital Partner for Academic Medicine," *Human Pathology* 28 (October 1997): 1117–22; Tinker Ready, "Market Research or Scientific Research? Study Raises Questions," *Raleigh News and Observer*, 16 April 1995, A25.

111 Quoted in Marshal, "Gene Therapy's Growing Pains," 1055.

112 Ibid.

113 "Biotechnology: Seeking Cures and Therapies for Children's Diseases," publication submitted to hearings by BIO (Biotechnology Industry Organization); "Research on Childhood Diseases by Entrepreneurs," *Hearing before the Committee on Small Business, United States Senate*, 26 May 1994 (Washington, D.C.: U.S. Government Printing Office, 1995), 80.

114 Gina Kolata, "Gene Therapy Shows No Benefit in Two Studies," *New York Times*, 2 September 1995, A24.

115 "Rates of transfer and expression vary dramatically in different patients." Marshall, "Gene Therapy's Growing Pains," 1052.

116 Quoted in Tim Beardsley, "Clearing the Airways," *Scientific American*, December 1990, 28–29.

117 Lawrence Fisher, "Bottling the Stuff of Dreams: Gains in Gene Therapy Encourage the Industry," *New York Times*, 1 June 1995, D1.

118 Andrew Pollack, "Gene Therapy's Focus Shifts, from Rare Illnesses," *New York Times*, 4 August 1998, F1.

119 Theodore Friedmann, "The Promise and Overpromise of Human Gene Therapy," *Gene Therapy* 1 (1994): 217–18.

120 Paul Martin and Sandra Thomas, "The Commercial Development of Gene Therapy in Europe and the USA," *Human Gene Therapy* 9 (1 January 1998): 87–114; Breffni X. Baggot, "Human Gene Therapy Patents in the United States," *Human Gene Therapy* 9 (1 January 1998): 151–57; Kathryn Brown, "Major Pharmaceutical Companies Infuse Needed Capital into Gene Therapy Research," *Scientist* 9 (13 November 1995): 1, 10. The latter article's subtitle reads, "Cautious observers note, however, that the fate of the new industry may hinge on a flurry of recently approved trials."

121 See glossary entry for ornithine transcarbamoylase (OTC) deficiency. Jesse Gelsinger had a form of OTC deficiency known as a "mosaic"

form, one that originated as a spontaneous mutation when he was in the womb and did allow his body to produce some very low levels of functional OTC.

122 Sheryl Gay Stolberg, "The Biotech Death of Jesse Gelsinger," *New York Times Magazine* 149 (28 November 1999): 136–40, 149–50, at 136–37.

123 Nicholas Wade, "Patient Dies in Trial of Gene Treatment," *New York Times*, 29 September 1999, A1, A24. The informed-consent paperwork presented to the Gelsingers leading up to Jesse's eighteenth birthday had been drafted with the help of the university's leading bioethicist, Arthur Caplan, and had been validated by the university's Institutional Review Board and approved by the FDA as well as by the independent federal advisory committee known as the RAC (Recombinant DNA Advisory Committee), which reports directly to the director of the NIH.

124 *Dateline NBC*, 20 September 2002, transcript.

125 Ibid.

126 Jesse's blood disorder produced an unfortunate cascade effect. As the red blood cells broke down, they liberated protein into the bloodstream. The protein, in turn, stimulated the production of ammonia, which Jesse's OTC-deficient liver was not capable of removing. These signs of liver failure were only the beginning.

127 The story is outlined in gripping detail in Stolberg, "Biotech Death of Jesse Gelsinger."

128 Leslie Roberts, "A Promising Experiment Ends in Tragedy," cover story, *U.S. News and World Report*, 11 October 1999, 43. See also Wade, "Patient Dies in Trial of Gene Treatment," A24, where Paul Gelsinger is quoted as saying, "The doctors were as devastated as I am. It was because of these men that I had my son for 18 years."

129 Among the defendants, the suit also named the University of Pennsylvania, two of its affiliated hospitals, and (in a novel twist) Arthur Caplan, the bioethics professor at Penn who convincingly argued to the Penn researchers that their trial should target relatively healthy, adult subjects with OTC deficiency. These subjects, he reasoned, were wholly capable of making an informed decision; they were less susceptible to exploitation than the sick infants and distraught parents who are victimized by the severest and most common form of OTC.

130 *Dateline* transcript.

131 A series of errors were attributed to Penn researchers in the wake of the FDA's initial investigation. First, although the informed-consent form

submitted to and approved by the FDA and the RAC did mention the fatal blood and liver complications suffered by monkeys in Penn's pre-clinical studies of the adenovirus, the informed-consent forms signed by the Gelsingers did not. This was an egregious omission, from the FDA's standpoint, especially in light of the fact that the day before his injection Gelsinger's ammonia levels had risen to a level that pre-cluded his participation in the experiment (according the protocol's own standards).

132 Julian Savulescu, "Harm, Ethics, and the Gene Therapy Death," *Journal of Medical Ethics* 27 (2001): 148–50.

133 These facts are outlined in Joanne Silberner, "A Gene Therapy Death," *Hastings Center Report*, March–April 2000, 6.

134 "Penn's Gene Therapy Director Stepping Down," *Gene Therapy Weekly*, 23 May 2002, 7–8.

135 Two gene therapy trials (on liver cancer and colorectal cancer) con-ducted by the Schering-Plough Company were halted by the FDA. See "Patient's Death Stops Gene Therapy Studies," *New York Times*, 12 Octo-ber 1999, A29.

136 Wilson explained, for instance, that Jesse's ammonia levels were ac-ceptable on the day of the injection. Sheryl Gay Stolberg, "FDA Offi-cials Fault Penn Team in Gene Therapy Death," *New York Times*, 9 De-cember 1999, A22.

137 Silberner, "Gene Therapy Death," 6.

138 *Dateline* transcript. A major factor in Gelsinger's turn against Wilson was the disclosure that Wilson's own animal studies had resulted in deaths, a fact never acknowledged by Wilson and the Penn research-ers until the investigations following Jesse's death. Those deaths were precisely the ones Wilson had the greatest duty to report during the consent process.

139 The actions of Wilson and the Penn researchers were investigated from every angle after Jesse's death, a path that ultimately led to a legal settlement between the Gelsinger family and the University of Pennsylvania (in 2000), a formal investigation of Wilson and Penn by the FDA (in 1999–2000), a restructuring of priorities and practices at Penn's Gene Therapy Institute (in 2002), and Wilson's dismissal as the director of the Gene Therapy Institute (in 2002). See "Penn Settles Suit on Gene Therapy," *New York Times*, 4 November 2000, A18; "Family Settles Suit over Death in Gene Therapy," *Wall Street Journal*, 6 Novem-

ber 2000, B6; Gretchen Vogel, "FDA Moves against Penn Scientist," *Science*, 15 December 2000, 2049–50; and "Penn's Gene Therapy Director Stepping Down," *Gene Therapy Weekly*, 23 May 2002, 7–8.

140 "Death at the Hands of Science," editorial, *New York Times*, 31 July 2001. At this point the gene therapy community began hastily to revise its claims and to recharacterize its studies, much as Crystal had done earlier. Researchers turned their attention to a new kind of scaled-down gene therapy, labeled "gene-assist therapies" because the goal was to deliver genes not to cells but to the proteins that regulate chloride transport. As one Associated Press story noted in July 1999, "Studies of three drugs called 'gene assist therapies' are in their early stages, experts caution. But if they work . . . patients could expect more normal lives by using a daily medicine to control a genetic defect that causes cystic fibrosis." Lauran Neergaard, "Early Studies Prompt Hope for New Way to Attack Cystic Fibrosis," Associated Press, 5 July 1999 (http://www.canoe.ca/Health9907/05_cf.html), accessed 11 July 2005.

141 Stolberg, "Biotech Death of Jesse Gelsinger," 138–39.

142 In mid-1995, on the advice of a panel of experts, NIH director Harold Varmus reduced the membership of the RAC from twenty-five to fifteen and stripped it of its approval authority. Varmus argued that in making this decision he was combating the overselling that was rife in the field of gene therapy. He later argued that he saw the RAC as doing its work ineffectively because it approved too many "troubling" protocols—that is, experiments that were not adequately peer-reviewed or conducted with the public interest in mind. In the words of Dr. Nelson Wivel (one of the RAC's former executive directors and later a colleague of James Wilson at Penn), "Some days . . . it felt as though the RAC was helping the biotech industry raise money. Dr. Varmus hated that." Others who wished to combat the overselling of gene therapy saw Varmus's actions regarding the RAC as self-defeating. For them, what was needed was better regulation, not less. As Stolberg noted in her *New York Times* article, Jesse Gelsinger's death confirmed the objection voiced by Varmus's critics, who saw his decision as allowing "gene-therapy researchers to ignore the panel and keep information about safety to themselves." Ibid., 139.

143 "AIDS politics [had] produced strange political allies. The antiregulation Reagan/Bush administration and the gay community probably had one interest in common: deregulating the drug approval process."

George Annas, "Faith (Healing), Hope, and Charity at the FDA: The Politics of AIDS Drug Trials," *Villanova Law Review* 34 (1989): 771–97.

144 There was more to the story. Drug research enterprises often perceived safety information as proprietary and resisted sharing it. The RAC confronted this problem of nondisclosure at its September 1999 meeting (before Jesse's death) when its members were presented with frank testimony from the Schering-Plough Company that information about side effects should be classified as a trade secret and with a sixteen-month-old letter (dated 14 May 1998) from Dr. Ronald Crystal of the New York Hospital and Cornell Medical Center asking that information about a patient death in one of his gene therapy trials be kept confidential. "The premise of the RAC review process from its inception was that all nonproprietary details about the protocol itself and all adverse events would be publicly reported," said Dr. LeRoy Walters, "and in a timely way." Sheryl Gay Stolberg, "U.S. Panel Moves to Force Disclosure in Genetic Testing," *New York Times*, 30 October 1999. In December 1999 a spokesperson for Schering-Plough, a company with several gene therapy trials in progress, commented that "immediate disclosure of adverse outcomes is bad science." See Rick Weiss, "Gene Therapy Firms Resist Publicity: U.S. Regulators, Researchers Are Divided on Releasing Information on Adverse Effects," *Washington Post*, 11 December 1999, A2.

145 Michael Schechter, Brent Shelton, Peter Margolis, and Stacey Fitzsimmons, "The Association of Socioeconomic Status with Outcomes in Cystic Fibrosis Patients in the United States," *American Journal of Respiratory and Critical Care Medicine* 163 (2001): 1331–37, at 1336.

146 Patricia Brennan, "His Daughter's Legacy: 'Alex, The Life of a Child,'" *Washington Post*, 20 April 1986, TV Tab, 5.

147 Leah Y. Latimer, "Arlington Nazi Says Party Plans Shift to Midwest," *Washington Post*, 25 December 1982, B1.

148 V. Scotet, D. Barton, J. Watson, M. Audrezet, T. McDevitt, S. McQuaid, C. Shortt, M. De Braekeleer, C. Ferec, and C. Le Marechal, "Comparison of the CFTR Mutation Spectrum in Three Cohorts of Patients of Celtic Origin from Brittany (France) and Ireland," *Human Mutation* 22 (July 2003): 105.

149 Rick Weiss, "The Good, the Bad, and the Unknown: Scientists Find That Some Genes Aren't Evil, They're Just Misunderstood," *Washington Post*, 11 October 1994, Z7.

150 Ellen Lee, "On the Front Lines against Cystic Fibrosis," *Atlanta Journal and Constitution*, 23 August 1998, 04C. See also Tim Friend, "Treatment of Cystic Fibrosis on the Fast Track," *USA Today*, 14 April 1998, D7: "CF is the most common fatal, inherited disease among whites, affecting 30,000 children and young adults in the USA."

151 Jane E. Brody, "Scientists Plot Tactics to Outmaneuver Cystic Fibrosis Gene," *New York Times*, 14 January 2003, A5.

152 Peg Meier, "Playing for Life," *Minnesota Star Tribune*, 1 November 1995, E1.

CHAPTER 3. A PERILOUS LOTTERY FOR THE BLACK FAMILY

1 Hugh Chaplin, *Lenabell: A Doctor's Memoir of a Remarkable Woman's Eighty Year Battle with Sickle Cell Disease* (Philadelphia: Xlibris Corporation, 2003), 176, 77.

2 James Jones, *Bad Blood: The Tuskegee Syphilis Experiment* (New York: Free Press, 1981); Susan Reverby, ed., *Tuskegee's Truths: Rethinking the Tuskegee Syphilis Study* (Chapel Hill: University of North Carolina Press, 2000).

3 See Keith Wailoo, *Dying in the City of the Blues: Sickle Cell Anemia and the Politics of Race and Health* (Chapel Hill: University of North Carolina Press, 2001). Today, scientists appear much more circumspect about using race as a marker of biological variation. Luigi Luca Cavalli-Sforza, who first began work as a population geneticist in the 1940s, has recently argued that the examples of sickle cell disease and thalassemia demonstrate not only the principles of the "heterozygote advantage" but also the impossibility of "racial purity" or a truly homogenous population. Luigi Luca Cavalli-Sforza, *Genes, Peoples, and Language* (Berkeley and Los Angeles: University of California Press, 2000), 46–49.

4 Wailoo, *Dying in the City of the Blues*.

5 Keith Wailoo, "Inventing the Heterozygote: Molecular Biology, Racial Identity, and the Narratives of Sickle Cell Disease, Tay Sachs, and Cystic Fibrosis," in *Race, Nature, and the Politics of Difference*, ed. Donald Moore, Jake Kosek, and Anand Pandian (Durham: Duke University Press, 2003), 235–53.

6 Wailoo, *Dying in the City of the Blues*.

7 Dr. Michael Blaese, chief of the National Cancer Institute's cellular immunology section, quoted in "Gene Therapy May Save Kids," *St. Petersburg (Florida) Times*, 18 May 1993, A1.

8 Bill Deitrich, "Genetics: Finding Genes Doesn't Assure Cures," *Seattle Times*, 6 April 1993, F1.

9 Stuart Edelstein, *The Sickled Cell: From Myths to Molecules* (Cambridge, Mass.: Harvard University Press, 1986). See also Simon Feldman and Alfred Tauber, "Sickle Cell Anemia: Reexamining the First 'Molecular Disease,'" *Bulletin of the History of Medicine* 71 (winter 1997): 623–50.

10 Linus Pauling, Harvey Itano, S. J. Singer, and Ibert Wells, "Sickle Cell Anemia, a Molecular Disease," *Science* 110 (November 1949): 543–48.

11 Keith Wailoo, "Detecting 'Negro Blood': Black and White Identities and the Reconstruction of Sickle Cell Anemia," in *Drawing Blood: Technology and Disease Identity in Twentieth-Century America* (Baltimore: Johns Hopkins University Press, 1997).

12 George Gray, "Sickle Cell Anemia," *Scientific American* 185 (August 1951): 56–59, at 59.

13 Wailoo, *Dying in the City of the Blues*.

14 Paul McCurdy quoted in Nancy Hicks, "Report of Treatment for Sickle Cell Anemia Evokes Guarded Optimism from Researchers on Disease," *New York Times*, 1 December 1970, 21. For the first report on urea, see Robert Nalbandian et al., "Sickle Cell Crisis Terminated by Use of Urea in Invert Sugar in Two Cases," *U.S. Army Medical Research Lab* 896 (17 September 1970).

15 "Discriminating Disease," *Time*, 21 December 1970, 41.

16 "Sickle Cell Cure—The Promise, The Peril: Urea Combats Crisis of Disease but Causes Dehydration," *Medical World News*, 8 January 1971.

17 Frank Gardner and Walter Seegers quoted in ibid. Reprinted in *Congressional Quarterly*, 8 October 1971, S167086.

18 Nancy Hicks, "Blood Cell Sickling Is Inhibited in Laboratory Tests," *New York Times*, 28 May 1971, 38.

19 Paul McCurdy and Laviza Mahmood, "Intravenous Urea Treatment of the Painful Crisis of Sickle Cell Anemia," *New England Journal of Medicine* 285 (28 October 1971): 994.

20 George Segel et al., "Effects of Urea and Cyanate on Sickling in Vitro," *New England Journal of Medicine* 287 (13 July 1972): 59–64. In a later letter one researcher pointed to the failure of urea in dramatic terms: "Not only were the crises not ameliorated but the diuresis produced within a 20-hour period was massive, leading to excretion of 12,000 to 22,000 ml of urine. If the treatment team had not been alerted to this pos-

sible fluid loss, the patients could have become acutely dehydrated."
Jerome Brody, "Treatment of Sickle-Cell Crises," *New England Journal of Medicine* 287 (21 September 1972): 616.

21 B. H. Lubin and F. A. Oski, "Oral Urea Therapy in Children with Sickle Cell Anemia," *Journal of Pediatrics* 82 (February 1973): 311–13.

22 Nancy Hicks, "Two Studies Discount Urea as Sickle Cell Treatment," *New York Times*, 28 May 1974, 52.

23 Gray, "Sickle Cell Anemia," 59.

24 Richard Nixon, "Health Message," 18 February 1971, *Congressional Quarterly Almanac* 27 (February 1971): 37A–38A.

25 Luis Barreras and Lemuel Diggs, "Sodium Citrate Orally for Painful Sickle Cell Crises," *Journal of the American Medical Association* 215 (1 February 1971): 768.

26 Paul Gillette et al., "Sodium Cyanate as a Potential Treatment for Sickle-Cell Disease," *New England Journal of Medicine* 290 (21 March 1974): 659.

27 Anthony Cerami and Charles Peterson, "Cyanate and Sickle-Cell Disease," *Scientific American* 232 (April 1975): 50.

28 "The dazzling demonstration of scientific amenities in these articles may divert the reader from serious defects," he wrote. He then criticized the urea trials for "seven critically important violations of our protocol." Robert Nalbandian, letter, "Urea and the Sickle Cell Crisis," *Journal of the American Medical Association* 229 (2 September 1974): 1285.

29 Paul McCurdy, letter, "Sickle Cell Crisis and Urea," *Journal of the American Medical Association* 230 (9 December 1974): 1386.

30 Statement by Senator John Tunney of California, *Congressional Record*, 8 October 1971, S16080.

31 Barbara Culliton,"Cooley's Anemia: Special Treatment for Another Ethnic Disease," *Science* 178 (10 November 1972): 590–93.

32 William Hines, "Sickle Cell Anemia: A Stylish Disease," *Memphis Commercial Appeal*, 11 November 1971, quoted in Wailoo, *Dying in the City of the Blues*, 193.

33 Linus Pauling, "Reflections on a New Biology: Foreword," *UCLA Law Review* 15 (1968): 269, quoted in Wailoo, *Dying in the City of the Blues*, 186.

34 I. M. Klotz et al., "Rational Approaches to Chemotherapy: Antisickling Agents," *Science* 213 (August 1981): 724–31; Thomas Maugh III, "Sickle Cell (II): Many Agents Near Trials," *Science* 211 (30 January 1981): 468–70.

35 C. M. Peterson et al., "Iron Metabolism, Sickle Cell Disease, and Response of Cyanate," *Blood* 46 (October 1975): 583–90; Samuel Charache and W. Gordon Walker, "Failure of Desmopressin to Lower Serum Sodium or Prevent Crisis in Patients with Sickle Cell Anemia," *Blood* 58 (November 1981): 892–96.

36 "Desickling Cells with a Kidney Machine," *Science News* 114 (23 September 1978); "Benzyl Esters as a Desickling Drug," *Science News* 117 (16 February 1980); Klotz et al., "Rational Approaches to Chemotherapy"; S. Takashima and T. Asakura, "Desickling of Sickled Erythrocytes by Pulsed Radio-Frequency Field," *Science* 220 (22 April 1983): 411–13.

37 Maugh, "Sickle Cell (II)," 470.

38 S. Charache and M. Moyer, "Treatment of Patients with Sickle Cell Anemia: Another View," *Progress in Clinical and Biological Research* 98 (1982): 73–82.

39 "Penicillin Found to Aid in Treating Cell Disorder," *New York Times*, 19 June 1986, A19. The article refers to M. H. Gaston et al., "Prophylaxis with Oral Penicillin in Children with Sickle Cell Anemia: A Randomized Trial," *New England Journal of Medicine* 314 (1986): 593–99.

40 "Seeking New Blood to Stop Sickle Cell" (profile of Dr. Clarice Reid), *Black Enterprise*, October 1988, 66.

41 C. H. Pegelow et al., "Experience with the Use of Prophylactic Penicillin in Children with Sickle Cell Anemia," *Journal of Pediatrics* 118 (May 1991): 736–38, at 738.

42 Zora Rogers and George Buchanan, "Bacteremia in Children with Sickle Hemoglobin C Disease and Sickle Beta+-Thalassemia: Is Prophylactic Penicillin Necessary?" *Journal of Pediatrics* 127 (September 1995): 353.

43 Ibid. The authors noted, "Careful evaluation of febrile episodes of all patients with SC disease is necessary regardless of the age of the patient or the use of prophylactic penicillin therapy." See also P. Applebaum, "Antimicrobial Resistance in *Streptococcus pneumoniae*: An Overview," *Clinical Infectious Diseases* 15 (1992): 77–83; I. R. Friedlander and G. H. McCracken, "Management of Infections Caused by Antibiotic-Resistant *Streptococcus pneumoniae*," *New England Journal of Medicine* 331 (1994): 377–82; and P. J. Chesney, "The Escalating Problem of Antimicrobial Resistance in *Streptococcus pneumoniae*," *American Journal of the Diseases of Children* 146 (August 1992): 912–16.

44 W. Wang, "Antibiotic-Resistant Pneumococcal Infection in Children with Sickle Cell Disease in the United States," *Journal of Pediatric Hematology/Oncology* 18 (May 1996): 140–44. See also P. J. Chesney, "Penicillin- and Cephalosporin-Resistant Strains of *Streptococcus pneumoniae* Causing Sepsis and Meningitis in Children with Sickle Cell Disease," *Journal of Pediatrics* 127 (October 1995): 536–42.

45 J. M. Falletta et al., "Discontinuing Penicillin Prophylaxis in Children with Sickle Cell Anemia: Prophylactic Penicillin Study II," *Journal of Pediatrics* 127 (November 1995): 689, 690.

46 R. F. Holcombe and J. Griffin, "Effect of Insurance on Pain Medication Prescriptions in a Hematology/Oncology Practice," *Southern Medical Journal* 86 (February 1993): 151–56.

47 L. Williams et al., "Outpatient Therapy with Ceftriaxone and Oral Cefixime for Selected Febrile Children with Sickle Cell Disease," *Journal of Pediatric Hematology/Oncology* 18 (August 1996): 257–61. See also J. A. Wilimas, "A Randomized Study of Outpatient Treatment with Ceftriaxone for Selected Febrile Children with Sickle Cell Disease," *New England Journal of Medicine* 329 (12 August 1993): 472–76: "When the randomized group were compared, outpatient treatment saved a mean of $1,195 per febrile episode . . . With the use of conservative eligibility criteria, at least half the febrile episodes in children with sickle cell disease can be treated safely on an outpatient basis, with substantial reductions in cost" (475).

48 Charache and Moyer, "Treatment of Patients with Sickle Cell Anemia," 81.

49 "Counterattack on a Killer—Blacks Fight to End Tragic Toll of Sickle Cell Anemia," *Ebony*, October 1971, 85.

50 On the phenomenology of pain, its resistance to objective study, and its cultural significance, see Mary S. Sheridan, *Pain in America* (Tuscaloosa: University of Alabama Press, 1992); Roselyne Rey, *The History of Pain* (Cambridge, Mass.: Harvard University Press, 1993); Elaine Scarry, *The Body in Pain: The Making and Unmaking of the World* (New York: Oxford University Press, 1985); and Martin Pernick, *A Calculus of Suffering: Pain, Professionalism, and Anesthesia in Nineteenth-Century America* (New York: Columbia University Press, 1985).

51 E. Vichinsky et al., "Multidisciplinary Approach to Pain Management in Sickle Cell Disease," *American Journal of Pediatric Hematology/Oncology* 4

(fall 1982): 328–33; Orah Platt et al., "Pain in Sickle Cell Disease: Rates and Risk Factors," *New England Journal of Medicine* 325 (4 July 1991): 11–16.

52 Orah Platt, "Easing the Suffering Caused by Sickle Cell Disease," *New England Journal of Medicine* 330 (17 March 1994): 783.

53 Elisabeth Rosenthal, "The Pain Game," *Discover*, November 1993, 54–57. See also Loch Adamson, "Sickle-Cell Patients Seek Respect," *Bronx Beat Online*, 6 November 1996, a discussion with researcher Ronald Nagel about the issues revolving around SCD pain management (http://www.columbia.edu/cu/bb/sickle.html), accessed 11 July 2005. Episodes of the NBC television series ER have also highlighted the blurring of the line between SCD patients and "drug addicts." See "You Are Here" (season 11, episode 177870), 5 May 2005, and "Obstruction of Justice" (season 4, episode 466359), 11 December 1997.

54 Rosenthal, "Pain Game."

55 "Seeking New Blood to Stop Sickle Cell," 66.

56 "Switch on Genes," *Newsweek*, 20 December 1982, 85.

57 "Genetic Fix: Turning on Fetal DNA," *Time*, 20 December 1982, 72.

58 A. Bank, D. Markowitz, and N. Lerner, "Gene Transfer: A Potential Approach to Gene Therapy for Sickle Cell Disease," *Annals of the New York Academy of Science* 565 (1989): 37–43, at 37.

59 Charles Whitten quoted in Marian Segal, "New Hope for Children with Sickle Cell Disease," *FDA Consumer*, March 1989, 14–19, at 19.

60 The first two statements by Charache appear in "Scientists Cite Gains on Sickle Cell Disease," *New York Times*, 28 November 1989, C1, C6. The third statement by Charache appears in Charles Marwick, "Sickle Cell Problems Continue to Challenge Medical Science, but Some Progress Noted," *Journal of the American Medical Association* 263 (1990): 493.

61 "A Switch for Sickle Cells," *U.S. News and World Report*, 23 April 1990; "Sickle Cell Breakthrough: New Drugs Quell Symptoms," *American Health*, May 1990, 16. See also "Waking up Genes: A Flavor Enhancer May Provide the First Treatment for Sickle Cell Anemia," *Time*, 25 January 1993, 23.

62 Griffin Rodgers, "Recent Approaches to the Treatment of SCA," *Journal of the American Medical Association*, 24 April 1991, 66.

63 E. P. Vichinsky and B. H. Lubin, "A Cautionary Note Regarding Hydroxyurea in Sickle Cell Disease," *Blood* 83 (15 February 1994): 1124–28.

64 Samuel Charache, "Experimental Therapy on Sickle Cell Disease: Use of Hydroxyurea," *American Journal of Pediatric Hematology/Oncology* 16 (1994): 62–66, at 66.

65 Charache quoted in Warren Leary, "Sickle Cell Trial Called Success, Halted Early," *New York Times*, 31 January 1995, C1, C7.

66 Ron Winslow, "Technology and Health: Sickle Cell Anemia Pain Curbed Dramatically by Drug, Study Says," *Wall Street Journal*, 31 January 1995, B6.

67 Griffin Rodgers and Alan N. Schechter, "Sickle Cell Anemia: Basic Research Reaches the Clinic," *New England Journal of Medicine* 332 (18 May 1995): 1372–73.

68 Samuel Charache, "Experimental Therapy," *Hematology/Oncology Clinics of North America* 10 (December 1996): 1376.

69 "Winning the Lottery: Odds Are against It," editorial, *St. Louis Post-Dispatch*, 2 May 1992, B3.

70 "Marrow Transplant Found to Be a Cure in Sickle Cell Case," *New York Times*, 20 September 1984.

71 R. B. Scott, "Advances in the Treatment of Sickle Cell Disease in Children," *American Journal of the Diseases of Children* 139 (1985): 1219–22.

72 R. E. Hardy and E. V. Ikpeazu, "Bone Marrow Transplantation: A Review," *Journal of the National Medical Association* 81 (1989): 518–23, at 518.

73 F. T. Billings, "Treatment of Sickle Cell Anemia with Bone Marrow Transplantation: Pros and Cons," *Transactions of the American Clinical and Climatological Association* 101 (1989): 8–19; Ronald Nagel, "The Dilemma of Marrow Transplantation in Sickle Cell Anemia," *Seminars in Hematology* 28 (July 1991): 233–34; E. Donnall Thomas, "The Pros and Cons of Bone Marrow Transplantation for Sickle Cell Anemia," *Seminars in Hematology* 28 (July 1991): 260–62.

74 Sergio Piomelli, "Sickle Cell Disease in the 1990s: The Need for Active and Preventive Intervention," *Seminars in Hematology* 28 (July 1991): 227–31.

75 Nagel, "Dilemma of Marrow Transplantation."

76 Ernest Beutler, "Bone Marrow Transplantation for Sickle Cell Anemia: Summarizing Comments," *Seminars in Hematology* 28 (July 1991): 263–67.

77 Thomas, "Pros and Cons of Bone Marrow Transplantation."

78 Nagel, "Dilemma of Marrow Transplantation."

79 Ibid.

80 Eric Kodish et al., "Bone Marrow Transplantation for Sickle Cell Disease," *New England Journal of Medicine* 325 (7 November 1991): 1349–53.

81 O. S. Platt and E. C. Guinan, "Bone Marrow Transplantation in Sickle Cell Anemia: The Dilemma of Choice," *New England Journal of Medicine* 335 (8 August 1996): 426–27.

82 Susan Miller, "A Cure for Sickle Cell?" *Newsweek*, 19 August 1996, 64. See also Curtis Rist and Cindy Dampier, "A Life Now Worth Living," *People*, 11 November 1996, 201–2.

83 Charache, "Experimental Therapy," 1375.

84 Richard Carter, "Insurance Coverage and Bone Marrow Transplants," *BMT Newsletter*, May 1994. See also M. C. Walters et al., "Barriers to Bone Marrow Transplantation for Sickle Cell Anemia," *Biology of Blood and Marrow Transplantation* 2 (May 1996): 100–104. The authors point out that "among 4848 patients less than 16 years of age . . . 315 (6.5%) patients were reported to meet protocol entry criteria for transplantation . . . [and in this eligibility, there was] wide variation among the [22] institutions . . . [Among the 315 eligible,] 128 (41%) had HLA typing performed, and of these 44 (14% of those meeting the criteria) had an HLA-identical sibling." See additionally W. C. Mentzer et al., "Availability of Related Donors for Bone Marrow Transplantation in Sickle Cell Anemia," *American Journal of Pediatric Hematology/Oncology* 16 (February 1994): 27–29.

85 Charache, "Experimental Therapy," 1375.

86 Mentzer et al., "Availability of Related Donors," 29.

87 "Although some knowledge may be gained from offering transplantation to patients with sickle cell disease," noted one group of researchers, "we suggest that the use of transplantation for patients with sickle cell disease is not primarily a matter of research." Kodish et al., "Bone Marrow Transplantation," 1353.

88 Bank, Markowitz, and Lerner, "Gene Transfer," 42. In the same year (1989) another senior researcher in the field looked "to the proliferating scientific energy and money going into gene therapy research for the payoff in sickle cell treatment," which he characterized as "the ultimate therapy." Charles Whitten quoted in Segal, "New Hope for Children with Sickle Cell Disease," 19.

89 David Nathan, "Clinical Care—Sickle Cell Disease: Past, Present, and Future," paper presented at the National Sickle Cell Disease Conference, "Keeping the Promise of Treatment and Cure," 19 September

1997, Washington, D.C. He continued, "Another problem is that one has to get the transfecting stem cells, and create real repopulating capacity." Only two years before, Nathan had published a triumphant assessment of the "tremendous accomplishments and potential of the American biomedical research enterprise," focusing on the story of a young boy with thalassemia. David G. Nathan, *Genes, Blood, and Courage: A Boy Called Immortal Sword* (Cambridge, Mass.: Harvard University Press, 1995).

90 Gail Ross et al., "Gene Therapy in the United States: A Five-Year Status Report," *Human Gene Therapy* 7 (10 September 1996): 1781–90. Between 1989 and December 1997, there were no clinical trials in SCD. In CF during the same period, there were nineteen worldwide (fourteen in the United States and five elsewhere). See *Human Gene Therapy* 8 (10 December 1997): 301–38.

91 Chaplin, *Lenabell*, 176.

CONCLUSION. DREAMS AMID DIVERSITY

1 Anderson quoted in Leon Jaroff and Hannah Bloch, "Keys to the Kingdom," *Time* 148, no. 14, Fall 1996 Special Issue, 24–29, at 28; Collins quoted in Jean Seligmann, "Curing Cystic Fibrosis? Genes Convert Sick Cells," *Newsweek*, 1 October 1990, 64.

2 Allen Buchanan, Dan W. Brock, Norman Daniels, and Daniel Wikler, *From Chance to Choice: Genetics and Justice* (New York: Cambridge University Press, 2000), 61.

3 Kaback quoted in Tim Cornwell, "Jewish Marriage Makers Embrace Testing for Genetic Disease," *London Guardian*, 6 March 1994, 27.

4 Max Weber, *The Protestant Ethic and the Spirit of Capitalism*, trans. Talcott Parsons (London: Harper Collins, 1991), 182. This edition was originally published in 1930. Weber's text first appeared as a two-part article in 1904–5.

5 Keith Wailoo, *Dying in the City of the Blues: Sickle Cell Anemia and the Politics of Race and Health* (Chapel Hill: University of North Carolina Press, 2001).

6 E. Donnall Thomas, "The Pros and Cons of Bone Marrow Transplantation for Sickle Cell Anemia," *Seminars in Hematology* 28 (July 1991): 260–62.

7 Frank Deford, *Alex: The Life of a Child* (New York: Viking, 1983), 32.

8 Carl Elliott, *Better Than Well: American Medicine Meets the American Dream* (New York: W. W. Norton, 2003).

9 Sheryl Stolberg, "Gene Therapy on Newborn Sets Medical Precedent," *Houston Chronicle*, 16 May 1993, 2; "Gene Therapy May Save Kids," *St. Petersburg Times*, 18 May 1993, A1; "Heading off Genetic Diseases in Their Infancy," *USA Today*, 18 May 1993, D1; Michael Drexler, "A Cure of Cystic Fibrosis? Rainbow [Children's Hospital] Cheers New Gene Therapy," *Cleveland Plain Dealer*, 16 October 1993, 1B.

10 Gerald Grob, *The Deadly Truth: A History of Disease in America* (Cambridge, Mass.: Harvard University Press, 2002).

11 Bill Dietrich, "Genetic Research Escalates — But Locating Flaws Can Be a Long Way from Curing Disease," *Seattle Times*, 10 April 1993, A6; Tim Radford, "Code of Conduct: The So-Called Homosexual Gene Highlights the Dramatic Advance in DNA Research. It Can Save Lives and Alleviate Suffering but It Also Poses Huge Ethical Problems," *London Guardian*, 21 July 1993, 2.

12 "Gene Therapy May Save Kids," A1.

13 Christopher Feudtner, *Bittersweet: Diabetes, Insulin, and the Transformation of Illness* (Chapel Hill: University of North Carolina Press, 2003); Steven Peitzman, "From Bright's Disease to End-Stage Renal Disease," in *Framing Disease: Studies in Cultural History*, ed. Charles Rosenberg and Janet Golden (New Brunswick: Rutgers University Press, 1992), 3–19; Richard A. Rettig and Norman G. Levinsky, eds., *Kidney Failure and the Federal Government* (Washington, D.C.: National Academy Press, 1991); Alonzo Plough, *Borrowed Time: Artificial Organs and the Politics of Extending Life* (Philadelphia: Temple University Press, 1986).

14 "Worcester Firm a Step Closer to Finding a Gene Therapy: Emerging Business," *Boston Globe*, 29 August 1993, 78; Victoria Griffith, "A Market That Could Spiral: The Commercial Opportunities of Gene Therapy Are Growing by the Minute," *Financial Times*, 1 July 1993, 20; Alex Barnum, "Biotech Startup Gets Genentech's Backing: South S.F. Firm to Take 20% Stake in GenVec," *San Francisco Chronicle*, 4 March 1993, D2.

15 Paul Donohue, "Gene Therapy Offers Promise in Future for Sickle Cell Anemia," *St. Louis Post-Dispatch*, 28 October 1998, E2.

16 Jay Ingram, "Tracking the Travels of a Gene," *Toronto Star*, 8 March 1998, F8.

17 "FDA Suspends Gene Therapy Work," *Pittsburgh Post-Gazette*, 4 May

2005, A6; Sharon Begley, "Why Gene Therapy Still Hasn't Produced Major Breakthroughs," *Wall Street Journal*, 18 February 2005, B1; Michael White, "Gene Genie Stays in Bottle," *Weekend Australian*, 20 November 2004, B12 (a review of *His Brother's Keeper*, a book about the hope and disappointments of gene therapy for a patient with amyotrophic lateral sclerosis); Robert Matthews, "Gene Therapy Is Just an Expensive Myth, Claims Scientist," *London Sunday Telegraph*, 31 October 2004, O8.

18 Robin Marantz Henig, "Genome in Black and White (and Gray)," *New York Times*, 10 October 2004, sec. 6, p. 47.

19 Quoted in John Pope, "Heart Drug Study Triggers Questions: Test Results Promising for African-Americans," *New Orleans Times-Picayune*, 16 November 2004, 1.

20 Henig, "Genome in Black and White (and Gray)," sec. 6, p. 47.

21 Andrew Pollack, "Drug Approved for Heart Failure in Black Patients," *New York Times*, 20 July 2004, C1. Sociologist Troy Duster argued that the marketing of the drug had begun with the idea of a study focusing on only one group, an idea that Duster saw as "flawed from the very beginning . . . You can't just do a study on a single group. That's basic statistics." Quoted in David Kohn, "Drug Combination Reduces Heart Failure Deaths of Blacks: Research Targeted by Race Stirs Ethical and Scientific Questions," *Baltimore Sun*, 9 November 2004, A1.

22 Quoted in Pope, "Heart Drug Study Triggers Questions," 1.

23 January W. Payne, "A Cure for a Race? Heart Drug Findings Set off Ethics Debate," *Washington Post*, 16 November 2004, F1.

24 Frank Harris III, "'Black' Drug for Heart Baffles the Mind," *Hartford Courant*, 15 November 2004, A9.

25 M. Gregg Bloche quoted in Pope, "Heart Drug Study Triggers Questions," 1. See also M. G. Bloche, "Race-Based Therapeutics," editorial, *New England Journal of Medicine* 351 (2004): 2035–37.

abortion. See **selective abortion** and **therapeutic abortion.**

adenovirus. Any of a group of DNA-carrying viruses that causes conjunctivitis and upper respiratory tract infections (the common cold). In their attempts at "gene therapy," scientists have attempted to alter adenoviruses (so-named because they were first identified in adenoid tissue) to deliver specific genes to diseased parts of the body. See **gene therapy.**

amaurosis. Partial or complete loss of eyesight, especially in the absence of externally perceptible changes in the eye.

amniocentesis testing. A medical procedure used for prenatal diagnosis of disease. A small amount of amniotic fluid surrounding a developing fetus is drawn out of the uterus through a needle inserted into the pregnant woman's abdomen. The fluid may be analyzed to determine the sex of the fetus or to detect genetic abnormalities. The procedure is usually performed in the sixteenth week of pregnancy. Contrast **chorionic villi sampling.**

antibiotic. An organic substance, such as penicillin or streptomycin, that destroys or inhibits the growth of pathogenic (infection- or disease-causing) microorganisms. Antibiotics are themselves produced from certain fungi, bacteria, and other microorganisms. An antibiotic that is effective against a specific or limited range of pathogenic microorganisms is called a *narrow spectrum antibiotic*. Conversely, a *wide spectrum antibiotic* is effective against a broad range of pathogenic microorganisms.

Ashkenazic Jews or **Ashkenazim.** Jewish people of originally Yiddish-speaking, Eastern European ancestry. The Ashkenazim are one of the major ethnic divisions among Jews, and their ranks are often said to include Jews from Germany, France, and Central Europe as well as Eastern Europe. Most Jews living in the United States are Ashkenazim. See also **Sephardic Jews.**

autosomal dominant inheritance. Pattern of hereditary transmission in which only one parent need pass the gene in order for the trait to express itself in the offspring. Thus, if a child receives a gene that is dominant (from either parent), he or she will usually manifest the trait. If that gene is abnormal, the child will have the disease. A child conceived by an affected individual has a 50 percent chance of inheriting the abnormal copy of the gene (or inheriting the disorder) and a 50 percent chance of inheriting the normal copy of the gene (or not inheriting the disorder). Autosomal dominant disorders can occur in multiple generations in a family or affect multiple family members in the same generation, and they never skip a generation. Except when there has been a new spontaneous mutation, every individual affected by a dominant gene disorder has an affected parent.

autosomal dominant disorder, gene, or **trait.** See **autosomal dominant inheritance** and **autosomal inheritance.**

autosomal inheritance. Pattern of hereditary transmission in which the expression of a trait is independent of the sex characteristics of the offspring. Humans have twenty-three pairs of chromosomes: twenty-two autosomes and one pair of sex chromosomes. Genes located on the autosomes can be dominant or recessive. Each parent passes only one copy of every gene to a child. By definition, autosomal disorders affect male and female offspring equally. Contrast **X-linked inheritance.**

autosomal recessive inheritance. Pattern of hereditary transmission in which both parents need pass the gene in order for the trait to express itself in the offspring. Thus, if a child receives a gene that is recessive (from one parent and not the other), there is usually no visible evidence of the trait. If that recessive gene is abnormal, it will not manifest as a disorder as long as the individual possesses another functioning copy of that gene. When both copies of the recessive gene are abnormal, the genetic defect will typically manifest as disease. Couples who both have an autosomal recessive defect face a 25 percent chance that their future child will have the disorder, a 25 percent chance that the child will be normal, and a 50 percent chance that the child will be a carrier (will have one normal gene, one abnormal gene). Tay-Sachs disease, cystic fibrosis, and sickle cell disease are all autosomal recessive disorders.

autosomal recessive disorder, gene, or **trait.** See **autosomal inheritance** and **autosomal recessive inheritance.**

beta-hexosaminidase deficiency. An enzyme deficiency associated with a wide range of disorders. The enzyme occurs in two forms, beta-hexosaminidase A and B. A deficiency of the former type, called a *Hex-A deficiency,* leads to Tay-Sachs disease. See **Tay-Sachs disease.**

blood-brain barrier. A natural barrier in the human body that prevents many substances present in the bloodstream from entering the brain (or affecting the central nervous system). Blood vessels throughout the body allow many molecules to cross through to tissue, but the dense construction of the vessels in the head guards against brain entry. Blood gases such as oxygen and small nutritional molecules can make it through this natural barrier. However, the barrier is designed to exclude toxins and other harmful substances from entering the brain's pristine nerve cell habitat. From a therapeutic perspective, the barrier also prevents many potentially beneficial substances from entering the brain. Enzyme replacement therapies and experimental gene therapies are among those treatments that must overcome the natural blood-brain barrier if they are to correct a genetic condition involving the neurological system (e.g., Tay-Sachs disease). See **enzyme replacement therapy, gene therapy,** and **Tay-Sachs disease.**

bone marrow transplantation (BMT). A procedure intended to replace diseased or damaged bone marrow with healthy bone marrow. Existing bone marrow is deliberately destroyed by high doses of chemotherapy and/or radiation therapy before the new marrow is implanted. The replacement marrow must come from the patient (as in the treatment of certain cancers), from an identical twin, or from a donor who is not an identical twin but whose marrow provides a biological match. Most bone marrow transplants involve donors who are not twins.

BRCA1 and **BRCA2.** Genes discovered in 1994 and 1995 that are associated with increased risk of breast cancer. Jewish women of Ashkenazic ancestry are often said to be at high risk for breast cancer because they have a higher incidence of BRCA1 and BRCA2 genes than the larger population of women. BRCA genes are autosomal dominant. However, the disease (breast cancer) manifests only if both copies of the gene are abnormal. Normally, BRCA genes regulate cell growth and suppress tumor cells. One need inherit only a single abnormal copy of a BRCA gene to be at increased risk for breast cancer and to be considered a carrier. Scientists have theorized that breast cancer occurs in a carrier of an abnormal BRCA gene when that person's other, otherwise normal, BRCA gene undergoes a mutation in the cell—at which point the individual's breast cell possesses no functional copy of the BRCA gene to suppress tumor growth. See **autosomal inheritance** and **autosomal dominant inheritance.**

carrier. In the context of genetic or hereditary diseases, someone who possesses a potentially disease-causing trait in his or her chromosomal DNA. In the case of autosomal recessive traits (like the genes for Tay-Sachs disease, cystic fibrosis, and sickle cell disease), carriers do not themselves have the disease. See **autosomal inheritance** and **autosomal recessive inheritance.**

cerebral sphingolipidosis. One among several lipid (fat) storage disorders. This disease affects the brain and is characterized by failure to break down sphingolipids (lipids synthesized in the golgi complex).

chorionic villi sampling (CVS). A prenatal test in which a catheter or thin needle is inserted into the womb to extract some of the chorionic villi (tissue from the developing placenta). The chorionic villi is composed of cells that develop from the same fertilized egg cell as the fetus, and thus shares the same chromosomal DNA as the fetus. CVS can be performed in a doctor's office or hospital between the tenth and twelfth weeks of pregnancy. Contrast **amniocentesis.**

Cooley's anemia. An inherited blood disease characterized by the absence of normal hemoglobin and by severe anemia, enlargement of the heart, spleen, and liver, and skeletal deformations. This disease is a form of thalassemia, sometimes called *thalassemia major*, and is usually fatal.

cystic fibrosis (CF). An autosomal recessive disease characterized by a cluster of symptoms including high levels of electrolytes in the sweat, pancreatic insufficiency, digestive problems, cirrhosis of the liver, infertility (in males), and an accumulation of thick mucus in the lungs accompanied by frequent infections and tissue scarring. There may also be damage to the right side of the heart because it is subjected to increased pressure as it attempts to pump blood through the damaged lungs. CF was originally called *cystic fibrosis of the pancreas*. See also **electrolytes, mucoviscidosis.**

DNA (deoxyribonucleic acid). The material in the nucleus of cells in all life forms that carries genetic information and is capable of replicating itself (and synthesizing ribonucleic acid, or RNA). DNA is constructed of two long chains of nucleotides twisted in a double helix and joined by hydrogen bonds. The sequence of nucleotides— adenine and thymine or cytosine and guanine—shapes an individual's hereditary characteristics.

electrolytes. Any of various minerals (such as sodium, potassium, or chloride) that carry an electric charge (ions) in blood, sweat, or other body fluids. Electrolytes are required by cells to regulate the flow of water molecules through the cell membranes.

enzyme replacement therapy. A way to treat a genetic abnormality by replacing the enzyme that the gene cannot produce. Genes are basically blueprints for proteins, and proteins are essentially enzymes. Thus, when a gene is defective, it fails to code for the protein (or enzyme) for which it is designed. The effect is that the enzyme will be defective or missing altogether. Among the most successful enzyme replacement therapies currently in use are those for cystic fibrosis (oral pancreatic extracts) and Gaucher's disease.

epithelial cells. Cells that cover the surface of the body and line its cavities.

Fanconi's anemia. A rare hereditary anemia characterized by retarded growth (hypoplasia) of the bone marrow and abnormally low levels of white blood cells, platelets, and erythrocytes in the blood.

gangliosidoses. A group of diseases caused by the deficiency of an enzyme necessary for the breakdown of lipids or fatty molecules (gangliosides). These deficiencies can produce devastating neurological symptoms. Tay-Sachs disease (a beta-hexosaminidase deficiency) is categorized as a GM2 gangliosidosis.

Gaucher disease or **Gaucher's disease.** A disease that has been described as the most common lipid storage disorder. It results from the deficiency of an enzyme (glucocerabrocidase) that normally helps the body break down specific fatty substances. The glucocerabrocidase deficiency allows these fatty substances to accumulate in the so-called Gaucher cells found in the bone marrow, spleen, liver, and other parts of the body. Once there, those fatty substances become toxic and can cause anemia, easy bruising and bleeding (low platelet count), bone pain, and bone fractures. The course of the disease is quite variable, ranging from no outward symptoms to severe disability and death. There are three types of Gaucher's disease. Type I is often said to be the most common genetic disorder found among Ashkenazic Jews.

Type I is also the mildest form of Gaucher's. It can emerge at any time from infancy to adulthood, and it does not affect the brain or have significant neurological symptoms. Type I is manageable using enzyme (glucocerabrocidase) replacement therapy. In contrast to Type I, the other two forms of Gaucher's involve severe neurological effects and strike in infancy (Type II) or childhood (Type III); in addition, their incidence is roughly the same across ethnicities. Enzyme replacement therapy has shown disappointing results in cases of Gaucher's with neurological involvement. The cause of the enzyme deficiency in all forms of Gaucher's disease is genetic, the result of a mutation received from both parents. It is an autosomal recessive disorder. See also **Ashkenazic Jews, autosomal recessive inheritance, Jewish genetic disorders,** and **lipid storage disorders.**

gene pool. The collection of genes of all the individuals in an interbreeding population.

genome. A single, complete set of chromosomes in an organism.

gene therapy. Experimental technology aimed at treating disease by attempting to replace a defective gene in the body with a healthy one. This can be done in many ways—for example, by removing bone marrow cells, then using genetic engineering techniques to change defective sequences in the DNA and reimplanting the altered cells. Other attempts at gene therapy have employed modified viruses (adenoviruses, retroviruses, etc.) as a delivery mechanism to attempt to carry healthy genes to a diseased part of the body.

gene transfer. A more technical term for *gene therapy* denoting the transfer of healthy genes to a diseased part of the body in the hope that the new genes will produce the protein normally required by the body, and thereby correct the problem.

genetic disease. A disease that is linked to genetic material either inherited from parents or present because of individual mutation. Thus, the term *genetic disease* overlaps with, but is not synonymous with, *hereditary disease.*

genetic screening and testing. Methods for determining whether a person has a specific gene, usually done to understand the likelihood that the person will develop a disorder or pass the disease to offspring. Genetic screening and testing takes many forms, including (1) carrier screening to see if an individual has a recessive gene mutation that he or she might pass to progeny; (2) diagnostic testing to see if an individual has a specific genetic disorder; (3) newborn screening to test an infant for congenital disorders; (4) predictive testing to determine the likelihood that an individual has a gene that might one day develop into disease; (5) prenatal testing to assess the health status of a fetus; and so on.

glycolipid. A fatty molecule (lipid) that contains one or more carbohydrate groups. Glycolipids are found in the plasma membranes of all animals and some plant cells. Blood group antigens, for example, are glycolipids.

graft-versus-host disease (GVHD). A condition in which bone marrow cells transplanted from a donor launch an immunological attack on the cells of the patient who received the transplant. GVHD can be treated with immunosuppressive drugs such as cyclosporin. Chronic or acute, GVHD can be a devastating, generally fatal, complication of bone marrow transplantation.

heart-lung transplant (HLT). A procedure, first performed in 1981, that replaces a recipient's diseased heart and lungs with organs from a donor. Recipients rely on long-term immunosuppressive therapy to slow the body's rejection of the donor organs.

hemoglobinopathy. A general term for a wide range of inherited blood disorders such as sickle cell anemia, hemolytic anemia, and thalassemia. These diseases are caused by abnormalities in the molecular structure of hemoglobin.

hemophilia. The oldest known hereditary bleeding disorder, in which the clotting ability of the blood is impaired and excessive bleeding results. Small wounds and punctures are usually not a problem, but uncontrolled internal bleeding can result in pain and swelling and permanent damage, especially to joints and muscles. Hemophilia results from a deficiency of clotting protein (either factor VIII or factor IX) and varies in severity depending on the amount of clotting protein that is missing. Hemophilia is caused by an inherited sex-linked recessive trait with the defective gene located on the X chromosome. It conforms to a classic X-linked inheritance pattern. Females are carriers of this trait. Fifty percent of the male offspring of female carriers have the disease, and 50 percent of their female offspring are carriers. All female children of a male with hemophilia are carriers of the trait. With very rare exceptions, only males have the disease. See **X-linked inheritance.**

hereditary disease. Inherited disease; disease passed from parent to offspring through genes.

heterozygote. A carrier of an autosomal recessive trait. In the case of autosomal recessive disorders like cystic fibrosis and sickle cell disease, the carrier does not have the disease but can potentially transmit it to his or her progeny. See **autosomal recessive inheritance.**

Hex-A deficiency or **hexosaminidase A deficiency.** See **beta-hexosaminidase deficiency** and **Tay-Sachs disease.**

human leukocyte antigen (HLA). A protein on the surface of cells that communicates to white blood cells whether the cells are "self" or "not-self." HLA enables the body's immune system to attack only invading organisms. HLA has been used in addition to ABO blood types to identify compatible donors for transplant procedures.

Huntington's chorea. A hereditary disease of the central nervous system that usually manifests at between thirty and fifty years of age, characterized by involuntary movements and progressive dementia.

hydroxyurea (HU). An orally administered drug that inhibits the synthesis of DNA. HU is used to treat chronic myeloid leukemia, sickle cell disease, polycythemia vera, melanomas, and cancers of the head, neck, ovary, and cervix. It may cause severe dehydration and kidney damage.

iatrogenic disease. Disease caused by medical treatment. The term encompasses a wide range of unintended complications of therapy, such as side effects or medical error.

Jewish amaurotic idiocy. The term used in the early twentieth century to refer to what later became known as Tay-Sachs disease. See **Tay-Sachs disease.**

Jewish genetic diseases. A term often used by medical geneticists and other interested parties to describe a group of inherited conditions that have an unusually high incidence among Jews of Eastern European (Ashkenazic) ancestry. In other words, the diseases are said to occur at much higher rates in this group relative to non-Jews and other Jewish groups (e.g., the Sephardim). The incidence rates can be as much as one hundred times higher for some conditions. There is no authoritative list of Jewish genetic diseases, but they include disorders that result from single-gene mutations (Mendelian disorders) as well as disease-predisposing conditions that result from a combination of genes. For Ashkenazic Jews, the Mendelian disorders include Tay-Sachs disease, cystic fibrosis, Type I Gaucher's disease, Canavan's disease, Fanconi's anemia, and at least eight others. Ashkenazic Jews are also known to have a high incidence of genes for the predisposing causes of colon cancer and breast cancer (in the case of BRCA1 and BRCA2). Sephardic Jews have normal rates of these diseases but a higher incidence of beta-thalassemia and a few other inherited conditions.

lipid storage disorders. A group of inherited metabolic disorders in which harmful amounts of fatty materials called *lipids* accumulate in the body's cells and tissues. People with these disorders either do not produce enough of one of the enzymes needed to metabolize lipids or they produce enzymes that do not work properly. Over time, this excessive storage of fats can result in permanent cellular and tissue damage, particularly in the brain, peripheral nervous system, liver, spleen, and bone marrow. The lipid storage disorders include Gaucher's disease, Niemann-Pick's disease, Fabry's disease, and Tay-Sachs disease.

lysosomal storage disorders. Disorders caused by dysfunctional lysosomes (minute saclike bodies, present in many types of cells, containing enzymes necessary for the process of intracellular digestion). Lysosomal storage disorders may result in cell damage and wasting, as in muscular dystrophy, or in the toxic buildup of undigested fatty molecules (lipids), as in the case of Tay-Sachs disease or Gaucher's disease. See **lipid storage disorders.**

mucopolysaccharide. A gel-like substance found in body cells, mucous secretions, and synovial fluids. Some genetic diseases (such as Hunter's disease) are called *mucopolysaccharidoses* because they are caused by a deficiency of enzymes for breaking down mucopolysaccharides. Such disorders lead to the accumulation of mucous material throughout the body, causing skeletal deformities, abnormal facial features, mental retardation, and decreased life expectancy.

mucoviscidosis. An early term for *cystic fibrosis*, highlighting the excessive mucus production throughout the body that characterizes this disease.

narrow-spectrum antibiotic. See **antibiotic.**

ornithine transcarbamoylase (OTC) deficiency. A treatable metabolic disease that impairs the liver's ability to rid the body of ammonia.

Like hemophilia, OTC deficiency is an X-linked disorder, meaning that, typically, women are carriers of the disorder while males are sufferers. OTC deficiency is the most common urea-cycle disorder. All urea-cycle disorders impair the liver's ability to remove ammonia from the body. Normally OTC is one of five enzymes that allow the liver to break down ammonia. The odds of OTC deficiency are calculated at 1 in every 40,000 births. It typically manifests in newborns, who within seventy-two hours can slip into coma as ammonia poisons their bloodstream, often leading to brain damage or death.

Orphan Drug Act of 1983. A federal law passed in the United States providing financial incentives to companies to develop drugs for rare diseases, in an effort to encourage research that would not ordinarily be profitable. The law provides a seven-year exclusive right to market to any company that develops the first drug of any type for rare diseases.

pancreatic deficiency. Inadequate production by the pancreas of insulin or digestive enzymes required by the body for cells to use energy from food.

pharmacogenomics. An emerging branch of pharmacology that explores how genetic factors influence the way organisms respond to drugs, and that seeks to tailor drugs to individuals based on their particular genome (or genetic profile).

physiotherapy. Physical therapy; treatment aiming to restore or maintain function and mobility, to relieve pain, or to mitigate permanent physical disabilities in patients suffering from disease or injury. Physiotherapy is employed in the treatment of cystic fibrosis, accidental injury, arthritis, low back pain, broken bones, heart disease, and some neurological disorders.

pneumococcal septicemia. Acute pneumonia affecting one or more lobes of the lungs caused by the bacterium *Streptococcus pneumoniae*.

polycythemia vera (PV). A blood disorder, also called *erythremia*, that involves the overproduction of red blood cells due to a disorder of the bone marrow.

postural drainage. A form of therapy often used in cystic fibrosis that consists of positioning a patient with the throat inclined downward and using percussion with the hands (striking the chest and back), taking advantage of gravity to help clear severe lung congestion.

prenatal testing. Testing a fetus in utero for the presence of disease prior to birth. See **amniocentesis testing** and **chorionic villi sampling.**

Pseudomonas aeruginosa. A species of bacteria that usually lives in soil, marshes, and coastal marine environments that may infect humans. It is rarely found in healthy individuals but tends to infect people with burns, those who have weakened immune systems, or those who are on respirators. It often spreads in hospitals. In patients with cystic fibrosis, the constant use of antibiotics to prevent lung infections related to excessive mucus production may allow pseudomonas to colonize the lungs, contributing to chronic pulmonary problems and early death. Pseudomonas infections may cause urinary tract infections, infections of the bloodstream, and pneumonia.

reductionism. The belief that all complex phenomena can be explained by breaking them down into component parts and isolating single causes.

sickle cell disease (SCD). An autosomal recessive disease, also known as *sickle cell anemia,* characterized by abnormal crescent- or sickle-shaped red blood cells. The sickled cells impair the oxygen-carrying capacity of the hemoglobin, depriving tissues of oxygen and blood. Because of their shape, the cells may also clog small blood vessels, causing severe pain and tissue damage. SCD may be experienced as acute pain in the joints, legs, or abdomen and may damage organs such as the liver, kidney, or brain. Lung infections are common.

selective abortion. The choice to terminate a pregnancy because the fetus is likely to be born with a serious birth defect or impairment. In this sense, selective abortion might be considered to be therapeutic (a form of treatment). However, the term has also been used to describe abortions in cases where a certain trait (e.g., the sex of the fetus) is simply not preferred by the parent. Such uses of selective abortion are generally not considered to be therapeutic. Contrast **therapeutic abortion.**

Sephardic Jews or **Sephardim.** Jewish people of Iberian (Spanish or Portuguese) ancestry. The Sephardim are one of the major ethnic divisions among Jews, and their ranks are often said to include Jews who migrated from the Iberian Peninsula to North Africa. See also **Ashkenazic Jews.**

strep (*Streptococcus*) infection/septicemia. One of several types of streptococcal (bacterial) infections in humans, which can result in pneumonia, skin infections, rheumatic fever, tonsillitis, scarlet fever, meningitis, and infected wounds. Pneumococcal septicemia (poisoning of the blood stream with virulent microorganisms) can be one of the severe complications of Tay-Sachs disease, sickle cell disease, or cystic fibrosis.

Tay-Sachs disease (TSD). A fatal autosomal recessive disorder of the central nervous system that results from the deficiency of an enzyme called *beta-hexosaminidase A (Hex-A)*, which normally helps the body break down specific fatty substances (GM2 gangliosides). The Hex-A deficiency results in the gradual destruction of the nervous system because the gangliosides become toxic as they accumulate in the brain and nervous tissue. There is no treatment for Tay-Sachs. Infants with Tay-Sachs develop normally for the first few months, then experience gradual and progressive mental deterioration followed by blindness, seizures, paralysis, and death. There is another, extremely rare form of Tay-Sachs that afflicts adults. People with late-onset Tay-Sachs have a similar mutation but suffer a more chronic form of the malady because they are able to produce some amount of the Hex-A enzyme. Both forms of Tay-Sachs disease have been categorized as GM2 gangliosidoses. See also **autosomal recessive inheritance, gangliosidoses,** and **lipid storage disorders.**

thalassemia. An inherited form of anemia, particularly prevalent in the Mediterranean, that involves impaired production of the red blood pigment hemoglobin. One form, beta-thalassemia, has an unusually high incidence among Sephardic Jews. See also **hemoglobinopathy.**

therapeutic abortion. The termination of a pregnancy out of concern for the health of the mother or fetus. A therapeutic abortion is usually justified on the following grounds: (1) to preserve the life of the mother; (2) to terminate a nonviable pregnancy; (3) to preserve the life of one or more fetuses in the case of a multifetal pregnancy; or (4) to prevent the birth of a child with defects associated with significant morbidity or mortality. Contrast **selective abortion.**

wide-spectrum antibiotic. See **antibiotic.**

urea. A water-soluble compound that is an end product of protein decomposition and is the main solid constituent of urine in mammals.

X-linked inheritance. Pattern of hereditary transmission in which the expression of a trait is dependent on the sex characteristics of the offspring. Humans possess twenty-three pairs of chromosomes: twenty-two autosomes and one pair of sex chromosomes. Males have X and Y sex chromosomes, receiving a Y chromosome from their father (which makes them male) and an X chromosome from their mother. Females have two X chromosomes, receiving one from each parent. A gene that is X-linked is physically located on the X chromosome. When someone has inherited a defective X-linked gene, that gene will manifest differently depending on which parent contributed that gene: sometimes it will produce disease, sometimes not. When a male inherits a defective gene, he will develop the disease because males have only one copy of the X chromosome; they thus have no backup copy to make the protein product that that gene would normally make for the body. Women who have one mutated copy of the gene are typically unaffected carriers because their one functional copy can produce all the protein product required by the body. For an example of an X-linked recessive inheritance disorder, see **hemophilia.** Contrast **autosomal dominant inheritance, autosomal inheritance,** and **autosomal recessive inheritance.**

Cystic Fibrosis Foundation, 36, 64, 71–72, 77–78, 91

deafness, 47–48
Deford, Alex, 68–69, 112
Deford, Frank, 36, 67–68, 73, 81, 112, 165
delta F 508 gene (DF508), 62–63, 111–12, 170, 196; and white identity, 62–63
Denmark, 62
diabetes, 63, 66, 87, 88, 92, 166, 167
Diamond, Jared, 25, 194
di Sant' Agnese, Paul, 68–71, 75
disease: symbolic significance, 1, 6, 10, 12–13, 15, 56, 58, 117, 121, 125. See also AIDS; beta-hexosaminidase deficiency; cancer; Cooley's anemia; cystic fibrosis; diabetes; end-stage renal disease; Fabry's disease; Fanconi's anemia; Gaucher disease; genetic diseases; graft-versus-host disease; heart disease; hemophilia; hex-a deficiency; Huntington's chorea; leukemia; lipid storage disorder; lysosomal storage disorder; malaria; muscular dystrophy; Orphan Disease Act of 1983; OTC deficiency; sickle cell disease; Tay-Sachs disease; thalassemia; tuberculosis
DNA, 97, 123, 142–43, 226–27
DNase, 98
Doershuk, Carl, 70
Dor Yeshorim, 3, 18–21, 28–31,

33, 40, 41–50, 52–59, 61, 63, 65, 120, 162, 163, 165, 192, 194; as genetic matchmaking, 41, 43–45, 50, 55–58, 118, 162, 189; origins, 18–19, 29, 189
drugs, 11, 31–32, 50, 52–55, 81, 83–87, 96, 98, 116, 134, 136–38, 139–40, 142–43, 147, 164–65, 171–72; cost, 53–55, 136–38, 146. See also antibiotics; BiDil; clinical research trials; cystic fibrosis, treatment options; DNase; enzyme replacement therapy; insulin; pharmaco-genomics; sickle cell disease, treatment options; Tay-Sachs disease, treatment options

Ekstein, Rabbi Josef, 18, 20, 29, 41–43, 46, 49, 51, 53–55, 189, 194. See also Dor Yeshorim
electrolytes, 227
end-stage renal disease, 167
entrepreneurs, 2, 5, 7, 65, 85, 89–91, 95–96, 100–102, 112, 118, 150, 157, 161, 162, 166, 169. See also capitalism
enzyme replacement therapy, 26–32, 40, 53, 57, 59, 64, 169, 227. See also Gaucher's disease, treatment options; Tay-Sachs disease, treatment options
epithelial cells, 227
ethical controversies. See genetic medicine, ethical controversies
ethicist(s), 10, 29, 44–45, 59, 154–55, 208–9
ethnicity and ethnic communi-

34; inheritance, 3, 17, 33, 117, 133, 224; issues of African-American identity, 6, 75–77, 114, 116–17, 121, 125, 130, 132, 164–65, 169 (*see also* thalassemia); legislation, 75–77, 113, 128; and malaria, 117; as molecular disease, 122–33; mortality, 4, 117, 124, 151; nature of malady as "blood disease" (hemoglobinopathy), 122–32; obscurity, 122–233; pain and crisis, 117, 121, 128–29, 132–34, 138–41, 145, 150–51, 158, 164; patient experiences and symptoms, 4–5, 12, 116, 119–21, 122, 124, 133–34, 138–41, 145, 146–47, 149, 154–57, 164; and pneumonia, 122; prevalence, 116; prevention, 134, 162; and racial politics/socioeconomic issues, 34, 75–77, 79, 117, 119, 121, 125, 128, 130–31, 138–41, 148, 153–56, 159, 164–65; and reductionism, 123–30; specialists, 116, 118–21, 122, 124, 130–31, 136–37, 140–41, 147–53, 156–57; symbolic significance, 1, 6, 10, 75–76, 117, 121, 125, 128, 132, 134, 138–41; treatment options, 5, 32, 118–20, 124–32, 134–35, 136–59, 161, 164–65, 213, 215, 219, 225, 230, 234; —antibiotics, 124, 134, 136–38, 141, 146, 215; —5-azacytidine, 142–44, 146; —bone marrow transplantation (BMT), 5, 12,

32, 119–20, 135, 141, 147–58, 159, 161, 164–65, 219, 225; —comprehensive care, 118, 130, 137, 149; —de-sickling agents, 124–25, 128–29, 131–32, 140, 213; —gene therapy, 95, 119–21, 141, 143, 158, 169; —hydroxyurea, 141–47, 156, 158, 230; —narcotic painkillers, 132, 139–41; —risks and side effects, 119, 120, 125–32, 135, 137, 139, 142–44, 146–57, 164–65; urea, 119, 125–32, 213, 234

Sickle Cell Disease Association, 158

Siegler, Mark, 29, 45

specialists and specialty groups, 4; adolescent medicine, 87, 204; cardiologists, 172; and cystic fibrosis, 12, 70, 72, 77, 80, 84–85, 90–91, 94, 100–102, 105, 108, 110–11, 118, 120–21, 123, 139, 147; family medicine, 72; "gene doctors," 95–103, 121, 125, 143, 157; geneticists, 8, 17, 20, 29, 61, 111, 163; hematologists, 4, 116, 122–23, 130, 135, 149–53, 157–58; molecular biology, 122–25, 127; neurologists, 4, 41; oncologists, 4, 158; pediatrician/pediatrics, 68, 84, 87; pulmonologists, 4, 66, 97; and sickle cell disease, 116, 118–21, 122, 124, 130–31, 136–37, 140–41, 147–53, 156–57; surgeons, 4, 85, 88–91, 111, 155; and Tay-Sachs disease,